Weight Lost Forever

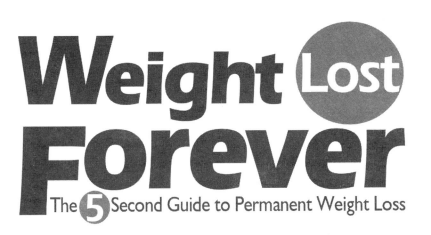

The **5** Second Guide to Permanent Weight Loss

Henry K. Chang, M.D.

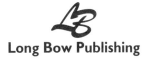

Long Bow Publishing

Published by Long Bow Publishing
P.O. Box 1360
Fair Oaks, CA 95628-1360
orders@longbowpublishing.com
www.longbowpublishing.com

Library of Congress Cataloging-in-Publication Data
Chang, Henry K.
Weight Lost Forever: The 5 Second Guide to Permanent Weight Loss
Includes Index

ISBN 0-9729368-0-7

For Sandy, the love of my life
And for our children Lisa, Denise and Philip

In memory of my father, William Chang
The greatest man I have ever known

Acknowledgements

I could not have written this book without the help of my wife, Sandy. She provided the crucial support I needed throughout this enormous undertaking. She also helped to modify my boring scientific style of writing into something that is more readable for the general public.

Many thanks to Bud Gardner and Jennifer Martin. Their encouragement and great advice were invaluable.

My special thanks to Duane Newcomb, whose guidance and editing account for this finished product that I am proud of.

Also, much credit to Deana Kuhlman for her creative design of the book and its cover.

Finally, my greatest and most profound thanks go to my patients, who put their faith in me and followed my program. This book could not have been written without their enthusiasm, dedication, and success in losing weight.

Patient Testimonials

These are comments from Dr Chang's patients who have benefitted from the Chang Method of daily weight monitoring and weight loss.

RE: Art Gallery Curator *(lost 30 pounds in six months)*

"I came to see Dr. Chang six months ago. I was discouraged because of continuous and gradual weight gain over the past ten years and concerned that the recent onset of menopause was adding to the problem. Tests showed I had no medical excuse, and Dr. Chang sat me down for a common sense talk about how to approach weight control for the rest of my life!

"His advice: find a good program like Weight Watchers and exercise two to three times a week or more. Most importantly, he recommended that I weigh in on a daily basis. He also advised me to set a moderate goal, reach it, then work at maintaining the plateau for awhile by monitoring my weight every day.

"I'm back, 30 pounds lighter, better fit than I've been in years—just in time to greet my 50th birthday this year. I'm still exercising and following Weight Watcher's awareness of daily food intake—minimum and maximum. And I'm not afraid of daily weigh-ins. They simply keep me on track and help me catch myself before my weight gets out of hand again. I enjoy being accountable and in control, not to mention just feeling awfully good in my clothes!"

DK: Driver Safety Manager *(lost 6 pounds in three months)*

"Several months ago I met my new doctor, Dr. Chang. I was a little apprehensive since I had packed on quite a few pounds over the last few years and my blood pressure was moderately high.

"Dr. Chang provided me with some clear information on achieving and maintaining weight loss. The doctor gave me three simple guidelines to follow:

- Eat no more than 40 grams of fat a day.
- Exercise for twenty minutes at least five to seven days a week.
- Weigh myself at the same time every day.

"By applying Dr. Chang's medical regimen I had significant decreases: blood pressure, weight, cholesterol, and bad cholesterol (LDL). I definitely feel a lot better. I have more energy and more confidence in myself to continue my new lifestyle changes.

"Thank you very much, Dr. Chang."

NB: Stockbroker *(maintained 75 pound weight loss for one year using the Chang Method)*

"After many, many years of failed dieting I became desperate. I was scared for my health, depressed with my appearance and very tired of not living a full and fun life. It doesn't matter how I lost my weight. Dr. Chang told me to use the scale every day. It is a great weight loss tool and will help me keep the weight off.

"For thirty years I had been told repeatedly not to get on the scale more than once a week and not to obsess with my daily weight fluctuations. This advice, no matter how well intentioned, was just plain wrong.

"As I came closer to my goal weight, the scale not only helped me recognize small plateaus, it also kept me motivated as the plateaus were broken. Getting on the scale each and every morning is now one of the many good habits I have developed over the last year. My weigh-in each morning puts me in control of my weight. I know immediately if my weight varies more than 1 pound up or down from my goal weight on any given day and I plan accordingly. I am accountable."

GA: Teacher *(lost 7 pounds in three months)*

"Seven pounds down—yeah! For years Dr. Chang has been telling me to weigh every day and eat no more than 35 grams of fat per day. I did the 35 grams on and off but didn't weigh every day. The weight got away from me while others encouraged me to, 'Oh, only weigh once a week. Why do that misery to yourself everyday?' Well, forget everyone else—now I weigh in every day and I have a handle on my own weight and life, and it's not misery. It's like a game. I now adjust my food intake accordingly. Thank you, Dr. Chang, for introducing me to this way of thinking. I'm hooked for life."

JW: Golf Professional *(lost 21 pounds in four months)*

"When Dr. Chang told me that to lose weight, I needed to weigh myself every day, I did not understand why. But after the first couple of months, the benefits were obvious. I lost 20 pounds. It was easy to see if what I was doing every day was helping me lose the weight. I will be weighing myself every day for the rest of my life. Thanks, Dr. Chang."

HL: Educator *(lost 22 pounds in five months)*

"I am a 58 year old woman who has battled obesity all of my adult life. I have been a patient of Dr. Henry Chang's for twenty years. Last spring while on a routine visit, we chatted about weight loss and exercise. At that time Dr. Chang said to increase my exercise. Since I recently had heart problems, he suggested cutting out the fats and slowly working on the weight. Then Dr. Chang said the key to losing weight was weighing every day.

"My immediate reaction was what does this healthy slim doctor know about weight loss? This was against all the diet programs that I had ever been on. And let me tell you, I have been on almost every imaginable diet. When I left I thought about what he had said and decided I would try it.

"I have lost over 20 pounds and it has been gradual and with little effort. I cut way back on meats and decreased fats and sugar. I do not count calories or points or how many of what foods I have consumed in a day. I just weigh every morning and it keeps me focused all day. I have recommended this to many of my friends."

OL: Retired *(lost 23 pounds in four months)*

"Stepping on my scale on a daily basis has helped me stay on a constant weight loss program and has helped me lose 23 pounds in a four-month period. In the past when I embarked on a dreaded diet, I only weighed once a week when I reported to the weight loss center. The stress associated with stepping on the scale was enormous and sometimes kept me from showing up. The daily weigh-ins help me adjust my eating immediately and when I attend my weekly weigh-ins I'm assured of my results. Thank you for the great suggestion to weigh on a daily basis. The results and compliments keep coming!"

HT: Engineer *(lost 29 pounds in eight months)*

"I started weighing myself each morning. I soon realized that what I ate the previous day had an impact on my weight. I then started reducing the amount of meat I ate and my weight began dropping, albeit very slowly. In four months I dropped 10 pounds. For the first time ever, I went through the Christmas and Thanksgiving holidays without adding weight. At no time did I feel I was on a diet, nor was I hungry."

Contents

Foreword

"Instead of fighting starvation as our ancestors did for hundreds of thousands of years, today we are faced with fighting obesity in a land of plenty. Ironically this fight may prove to be more difficult because our bodies have been programmed to covet food and to endure starvation, not excess. Dr. Chang's efforts and success in achieving weight loss in his patients comes at an opportune time due to the epidemic of obesity in this country and is a striking example of the impact that a single clinician can have when facing his/her patients with weight problems.

"An approach that emphasizes constant surveillance seems more logical to me than a crash diet over a short period of time. Dr. Chang has developed an innovative method of weight loss that is easy to understand, simple to follow, and effective. This book not only helps people to lose weight but also shows them how to keep it off."

Thomas A. Depner, M.D.
Professor of Medicine
University of California, Davis

Preface

As an internist who has been practicing medicine in the Sacramento area of California for over twenty-six years, I am pleased to see that statistics show we are a healthy nation. This is reflected by the increase in American longevity. I can attest to this by the number of my patients who are in their 80s and 90s. This increase is in part due to the tremendous advances in medicine. Some of these advances include better diagnostic tools such as CT and MRI scans, ultrasound tests, and endoscopic procedures, which help to diagnose diseases early at treatable stages.

There have been tremendous advances in medications, which are easier to take and are much more effective than before. Surgical techniques have also improved considerably, especially the less invasive procedures such as arthroscopies, laparoscopies, and balloon angioplasties. Unfortunately, most of these advances are expensive and are not always affordable or available to everyone.

We must not ignore the role of public health in promoting healthy Americans. I contend that some of the simpler, less expensive and not always medically-related changes have done more to keep us healthy than anything else. I am referring to the improved sanitation due to flush toilets, the refrigeration of foods, handwashing, sterile gloves, and sterilized surgical instruments. Also, immunization has effectively wiped out many diseases and saved lives.

There is one thing, however, that threatens this positive trend. That thing is obesity. Obesity has reached a catastrophic level in the United States. In fact, during the time I was writing this book, I had to revise the rate of overweight Americans from 56% to 65%.

It is unimaginable that one-third of our adult population is overweight and another one-third is actually obese. This rate is continuously increasing in spite of the fact that Americans spend over $30 billion annually on diet products. We can safely say that obesity has reached epidemic proportions. The scary thing is that there has been no solution to counteract this. I am afraid that if this trend continues we will soon be a very unhealthy nation.

During my years of practicing medicine, I have developed an innovative method to fight obesity that is over 90% successful for my patients. It does not involve a new diet, just a change in the way they approach losing weight. I would like to share this method with you and I hope that you will share it with your friends, so that we can spread the Chang Method to as many people as possible.

Introduction

I have always enjoyed taking care of patients when they are sick. More than that, I really like keeping them healthy. This means a healthy diet, regular exercise, and for overweight people, losing weight. These are natural ways to stay healthy. I have preached diet, exercise and weight loss to my patients at almost every visit for over 26 years.

Unfortunately, until this last year, I had not been very successful in motivating my patients to lose weight despite my intense efforts. I estimate that less than 5% of those patients succeeded in losing weight and maintaining weight loss. Then I discovered the weight loss program that involves daily weight monitoring. Since then I have used this program on 140 patients and have achieved an over 90% success rate. I was frankly quite surprised by this incredible success! I was even more surprised by the overwhelming enthusiasm my patients felt (and continue to feel) about my method, as reflected by their testimonials found in this book. Let me share with you how I came upon this daily weighing program.

I have been pretty lucky with my own weight for many years. I was able to eat whatever I wanted and never gained a pound. I also seldom weighed myself. The main reason for this was that I was an avid tennis player. I played tennis vigorously for a couple of hours twice a week. I also did some martial arts. Unfortunately, I injured my shoulder in martial arts and had to quit both sports. About a year later, I noticed that my pants were feeling rather tight. One day I looked sideways in the mirror and saw the unflattering sight of my protruding abdomen. I could not believe what I saw. I got on the scale and found that I had gained over 10 pounds!

I told my wife Sandy about my shocking discovery. She told me that she had noticed my weight gain and assumed that I had noticed it too. I got upset and unjustly blamed her for not telling me earlier. I soon realized that the fault was entirely mine for not monitoring my own weight. I then started to watch my food intake more carefully, exercise regularly, and weigh myself daily.

I have since lost all the excess weight I gained and have maintained this weight loss for ten years now. However, this has not been easy. My body always seems to want to gain those 10 pounds back whenever possible. I can only keep my weight down by monitoring it on a daily basis.

I have also observed through the years that most of my patients who maintained long-term weight loss weigh themselves frequently. From this, the idea of daily weighing was born.

As you know, virtually all of the weight reduction programs discourage people from weighing themselves daily. Let me reassure you that daily weighing *does* indeed work for my patients. However, in order for it to work for you, you must closely follow my instructions that are detailed in Chapter 2.

Chapter 1
Obesity And Its Detrimental Effects

Obesity is rampant in America. It is estimated that 34% of the adult population is overweight, and another 31% is obese, and those figures have increased by more than 75% since 1980! Obesity is associated with cardiovascular disease, diabetes, high blood pressure, strokes, gallbladder disease, osteoarthritis, sleep apnea, respiratory problems, and some types of cancer.

In the last few years, we have also discovered a condition that is associated with obesity called *metabolic syndrome*. This syndrome is defined as having at least three of the following five abnormalities: high blood pressure, high blood sugar, high blood levels of triglycerides, low blood levels of HDL ("good") cholesterol, and abdominal obesity (defined on page 2).

Metabolic syndrome is dangerous because it significantly increases the incidence of heart disease and strokes. Unfortunately, this syndrome is very common and affects 15% to 20% of our adult population. Obesity is the single most important factor in the cause of this syndrome. This means that to treat this syndrome you must reduce your weight.

● Overweight and Obesity Defined

Now let's define *overweight* and *obesity*. Today we use a measurement called body mass index (BMI) to determine if an individual is overweight or obese. This index is simply a ratio of weight to height. But the calculation is complex. We calculate the BMI by dividing one's weight in pounds by the square of one's height in inches, and multiplying the result by 703. See what I mean? You can find websites on the Internet that will calculate this for you. The Calorie Control Counsel website is a good one. Check this out at www.caloriecontrol.org/bmi.html

You are considered overweight if your BMI is 25 or more. We define obesity as a BMI of 30 or more and extreme obesity as a BMI of 40 or more. I find the BMI calculation too complicated for most people. We'll use something easier in this book.

● Abdominal Obesity

I prefer to use waist circumference to define obesity (called abdominal or central obesity). You are obese if you are a male with a waist circumference of over 40 inches, or a female with a waist circumference of over 35 inches.

Always take this measurement at the navel level. I once asked an overweight patient what his waist circumference was and he confidently told me it was 38 inches. I was surprised. I then took out my tape and measured his waist circumference and found that it was actually 44 inches.

It turned out that he wore size 38 pants but, like many obese people, he wore his pants at the level of his hips below his massive protruding abdomen.

Abdominal obesity is much easier to measure than the BMI. It is also an important measurement because fat in the abdomen is much more harmful to the body than fat in the arms and legs. This is due to the fact that abdominal fat is more metabolically active and makes free fatty acids and glycerin, which block the body's ability to take up glucose and also cause the liver to make more fats such as triglycerides. These all contribute to the development of heart disease.

• Diabetes and Obesity

Diabetes is also associated with obesity and is caused by an insufficient amount of insulin. As a result, the blood glucose rises. Diabetic patients have a much higher risk of cardiovascular complications than the general population. These include heart attacks, strokes, and poor circulation to the extremities, which may lead to gangrene and amputation.

To illustrate the devastating effects of diabetes, I

recall a young patient of mine named Debbie who was in her early 20s. (All names of patients in this book have been changed to assure patient confidentiality.) She had childhood onset diabetes and had been on insulin shots since she was 3 years old.

Debbie did not let her chronic medical condition interfere with her life. She went to school like everybody else and graduated from high school with top honors. She volunteered in the hospital as a candy striper while she was still in high school. She was cheerful and compassionate and was well loved by the patients, especially kids with diabetes. She was a ray of sunshine in the often gloomy hospital wards. Debbie went on to college after high school and was studying to be a physical therapist.

One day Debbie noticed increasing difficulty breathing. She ignored this for a couple of days thinking it was just a cold. She finally was so sick that she had to be transported to the hospital by ambulance. Unfortunately, she had a massive heart attack and had fluid in her lungs as a result of it. We treated Debbie with everything we had but were unable to save her. I was devastated. I kept wondering why would this happen to such a wonderful person at such a young age? Sadly, Debbie had no way to prevent her diabetes because she had juvenile-onset diabetes. However, many adults *can* prevent this terrible disease by reducing obesity.

Diabetic patients are also subject to complications that include kidney failure, retinal disease that can lead to blindness, and disorder of the nerve endings in the extremities.

In fact, the most common cause of kidney failure requiring dialysis in this country is diabetes. I recently lost a patient with diabetes who was on kidney dialysis. George was in his late 60s and had been suffering from diabetes for many years. He developed progressive kidney failure about five years ago. I recommended kidney dialysis at that time but he was resistant to the idea. Finally, his symptoms—including nausea, shortness of breath, weakness, and general malaise—were so severe that he gave in.

George immediately felt better on dialysis. However, he had to go to the dialysis center three times a week. At each dialysis session, all of the blood in George's body went through the dialysis machine, which took three to four hours. He would often feel weak and exhausted at the end of each session. Trips out of town required a tremendous amount of planning. He would have to arrange for kidney dialysis in a strange new place ahead of time, provided that there was a dialysis center nearby.

To add insult to injury, George's graft, an artificial connection between the artery and the vein in his forearm where the dialysis needle enters, would get infected from time to time. This would make him sick, and he often required hospitalization. Although dialysis saved him, George's life was full of restrictions and suffering. Over the last five years he gradually deteriorated. He was getting so weak that he could hardly walk. His heart began to fail. George declined any treatment for his heart and recently passed away. As you can see, diabetes shortens our lifespan and adversely affects our quality of life.

● Is Diabetes Inherited?

My patients often ask if heredity is the most important factor in determining whether or not they may be prone to becoming a diabetic. Heredity is definitely important, but it is not the only thing that causes diabetes.

Let me introduce you to the Pima Indians of Arizona and northern Mexico. They are genetically highly prone to diabetes. Those living in Arizona have an exceedingly high rate of diabetes of about 50% by the age of 50. However, the Pima Indians in northern Mexico, who are genetically similar, have a normal rate of diabetes. The reason? The Pima Indians in Arizona are, on average, 60 to 65 pounds heavier than the Pima Indians in northern Mexico. Because of this example and many others, it is believed that obesity is one of the most important factors for developing diabetes. I will discuss diabetes in greater detail in Chapter 5.

The good news about diabetes is that often weight loss can reverse its effects. Fortunately, you don't have to lose much weight to accomplish this. One of my diabetic patients lost 6 pounds; his blood sugar dropped to a normal range and he was no longer diabetic. Another lost 20 pounds and had the same positive result. I have many other patients with similar experiences.

In the next few chapters I am going to show you how to successfully fight obesity. It has worked for my patients—it can work for you.

Chapter 2
Intoducing the Chang Method

It is difficult to lose weight. It is even harder to maintain weight loss. It is estimated that over 95% of the people who lose weight gain it back. Many even overshoot their original weight. If you have gone through this, you know how devastating the yo-yo effect is. It is as if you have a thermostat inside set at your highest weight. The thermostat will eventually bring your body back to your highest weight, no matter how long it takes.

To add insult to injury, there is a tendency for all of us to gain weight as we get older. The thermostat then resets itself at the newer higher weight, so weight reduction is truly an uphill battle all the way.

● Winning the War

How can we ever win this seemingly hopeless war? The obvious answer is diet and exercise. However, this is not the whole answer. First, we need to understand how obesity occurs. When energy intake exceeds energy expenditure, the body stores the excess calories as fat. When this happens over a period of time we become obese. Energy intake is simply the amount of food we eat. Energy expenditure is more complicated. It has three components: (1) basal metabolic rate (BMR), (2) exercise-induced thermo genesis (or the amount of calories burned by exercising), and (3) the thermic response to food, which is the energy it takes to absorb, digest, metabolize and store food.

Of the three components, the number of calories burned by exercise is the only one we can easily control. This accounts for about 20% of our daily energy expenditures. In order to lose weight, we need to reverse the process. That is, we need to have energy expenditure exceed energy intake.

Increasing energy expenditure is achieved by exercise, which I will discuss in Chapter 4. Decreasing energy intake is achieved by dieting, medications and, in rare cases, surgery. Medications and surgery have many potential risks and side effects and should be tried only under close medical supervision. I will discuss dieting in Chapter 3.

Do diet and exercise work well for taking off weight and keeping it off? To answer that question, you just need to look at the number of diets and dieting programs as well as gyms and health clubs available. You can't watch TV without being bombarded by ads for dieting programs and dieting supplements. Ask obese people if they have tried to take off weight and most have a sad story to tell of one failed dieting attempt after another.

Regrettably, this has happened to many of my patients and friends. One particular example is a friend and patient of mine named Andre. Andre is a tall man who is also overweight. He has tried many types of weight reduction programs, his favorite being the Pritikin Program. He would go to the Pritikin Longevity Center for a few weeks and lose 20 to 30 pounds. However, he would invariably gain it all back in a matter of months after returning home.

Another example is a friend of mine whom I will call Paul. Paul is a very big man, both tall and overweight. One day I ran into him and noticed that he seemed thinner. I asked him if he had lost some weight. He seemed a bit annoyed by the question and answered that indeed he had lost some weight—100 pounds to be exact. I felt a little embarrassed but went on to ask him how he did it. It turned out he had been on a fruit and water diet for close to a year. I congratulated him and told him I was very happy for him.

Unfortunately, Paul gained back all of the 100 pounds in just a few months. He actually repeated this behavior by losing 100 pounds several years later. Sure enough, the end result was the same. Paul is now at his highest weight ever, even though he has lost altogether over 200 pounds.

When you stop to think about it, you will realize

that there must be a third element in addition to diet and exercise that is vital to maintaining weight reduction. The third element is **every day weight monitoring**. The heart of my program then is: (1) selecting a diet plan that works for you, (2) exercising at least twenty minutes a day, and most importantly (3) **monitoring your weight every day.**

Before I discuss my daily weighing program, let me share with you what Eva, a yo-yo dieter patient of mine, wrote: "I have been dieting for fifty years, sometimes very successfully, but I always gained the weight back. I am a good example of a yo-yo dieter. Dr. Chang's daily weighing has been a success for me because it puts me in control. It is a lot easier to lose 1 pound than 5. I have learned which foods make me gain and also retain water. It seems to make me more conscious of every thing I put in my mouth. Here's to more weight loss."

• Monitor Your Weight Every Day

Some experts claim that daily weighing is demoralizing, unnecessary and meaningless. Day-to-day variations in weight, they say, simply reflect fluid retention rather than actual weight gained or lost. They also insist that weight reduction is a gradual process that takes place over weeks or months rather than over days.

This is a big misconception. My patients often tell me they don't have to monitor their weight. They think they can tell what their weight is by how well or how poorly their clothes fit.   I find this method grossly inaccurate. By the time people can't fit into their clothes, they may have gained 10 to 20 pounds!

Based on my experience with treating overweight patients, I have learned that daily weighing is absolutely essential to losing weight and maintaining weight loss. In my program, the Chang Method, it is important that you closely follow the steps I will outline for you. If you do this, you will not be demoralized or discouraged. Instead, you will be in control and you will feel successful throughout the program.

● The Weight Maintenance Mode

The first step in the Chang Method is not weight reduction but weight maintenance. You can accomplish this through daily monitoring. Here are some instructions.

1. **Be sure you have a reliable scale**. Your scale doesn't have to give the same results as the scale in your doctor's office. However, the scale must be consistent. In other words, if you step on it three times it should give you the same reading. Lean left, lean right—it should show the same weight.

2. **Weigh yourself exactly once a day at the same time each day**. For example, weigh yourself in the morning before breakfast or at night before bed, without clothing. It would be meaningless to weigh yourself before breakfast one day and after lunch the next.

You have now started what I call the **Weight Maintenance Mode**. In the maintenance mode you tell yourself that you will not allow your body to gain any more weight. Success is defined as holding your weight and not gaining. *You do not have to lose weight to feel successful in this mode!*

As you weigh yourself every day, you may occasionally find yourself gaining a pound or two from one day to the next. Keep in mind that it is not a pound of fat you have gained. It is not possible to gain a pound or two of fat in one day. It takes much longer than this to gain fat.

This small amount of weight gain can easily be due to fluid retention, overeating, or eating too much salt. It really does not matter what the cause of the weight gain is. The point is it signals that your weight is heading in the wrong direction.

Do not be discouraged or demoralized by this small weight gain. Simply tell yourself that you need to reverse the trend and bring the weight back down over the next few days, either by eating less or exercising more or both.

It may take one day or it may take several days to restore the baseline weight. Be patient. Do not get discouraged. It is also important to avoid weighing yourself more than once a day. This would be nonproductive and meaningless because you are not comparing yourself under the same conditions with respect to the intake of food. Just continue to weigh yourself once a day until you stay relatively the same weight over a period of time. I recommend that you do this for about a month, or until you get the hang of it.

This **Weight Maintenance Mode** is relatively easy to do, especially for those of you who are at your highest weight. Some of you can probably maintain your weight without ever weighing yourselves. However, I ask you, how many of you were lighter ten or twenty years ago? I venture to guess that if you are like the patients in my practice, many of you were quite a bit lighter then.

I have a patient who is 39 years old. She has been gaining weight steadily for the past six years, since the birth of her last child. Now she is 30 pounds heavier than she was six years ago. Another patient is a 67-year-old retired mailman. Since retiring five years ago, he has gained 25 pounds because he no longer walks several miles a day delivering mail.

One more example is a young man who is 32 years old. He has been my patient for eleven years. Over that period of time he gained 50 pounds! Unfortunately, these are common examples of what happens to your weight over time.

Now consider this: if you started weighing yourselves daily and got on the **Weight Maintenance Mode** ten to twenty years ago, you would not have gained any weight over that period of time. This is the reason that even young people who are not yet overweight should get on the **Weight Maintenance Mode** to prevent future weight problems.

How long do you stay on the **Weight Maintenance Mode**? The answer is *forever*. This should become a life-long habit, somewhat analogous to brushing your teeth. Remember, success is defined as not gaining any weight. Give yourself a lot of credit if you have accomplished this. You do not have to lose weight to feel successful during this mode.

After you feel comfortable with the **Weight Maintenance Mode**, (e.g., after a month or so) you are now ready to start the **Weight Reduction Mode**. This obviously is harder than the maintenance mode.

● **The Weight Reduction Mode**

To achieve success in this mode you will need to eat less, exercise more, or both. Of course, you can't live this way the rest of your life. But you can do it for a while and then switch back to the maintenance mode to keep from regaining the weight you have lost.

Here is the approach that I want you to follow. Set for yourself the goal of losing 5 pounds over the next month. Tell yourself that this will be unpleasant. You will frequently need to go hungry and to exercise when you don't feel like it. However, realize that this suffering is only temporary. Say to yourself, "I can sacrifice for a month so that I can enjoy a better, healthier life for the rest of my life." If you have done this in the past, you can do it now.

Once you have succeeded in losing the 5 pounds over the month, give yourself credit for reaching your goal. Keep in mind that the body has a strong tendency to gain these 5 pounds back, whether it takes a week, a month, or a year. Remember the thermostat analogy—how it always wants to go back to the pre-set temperature. However, this will not happen because you will stay on the **Weight Maintenance Mode**, weighing yourself once a day. If you find yourself gaining 1 of the 5 pounds back one day, you will work hard on the subsequent days to take that pound off. Now you are 5 pounds lighter, forever!

Can you get by weighing yourself once a week instead of once a day? The answer is "no," because most of us can easily gain 5 pounds in a week and immediately nullify all the hard work it took to lose the 5 pounds. My patient, Gloria, who believes that weighing yourself once a week is not enough, wrote: "I lost 50 pounds on Weight Watchers. I've been at my goal weight for four months and feel that by weighing myself daily I am more in control. If I weighed myself once a week, I could easily gain 5 pounds. If my weight is more than 2 pounds above my goal, I immediately decrease my points the next day."

What about weighing yourself every other day? The problems with this are: (1) You can gain twice as much weight in two days than in one, which of course makes it harder to get rid of it, and (2) It is difficult to remember whether you weighed yourself yesterday or was it the day before? It is much easier to just get into the routine of weighing yourself once a day, like brushing your teeth.

Finally, some patients tell me that they weigh themselves almost every day. This reminds me of the joke about the man who told his friends that he had sex with his wife "almost every day." He almost had sex with her on Monday, almost on Tuesday, almost on Wednesday, and so on.

By following the above daily weighing program, you can lose 5 pounds and keep it off for the rest of your life. As you will see from a study on how to prevent diabetes that I will describe in Chapter 5, you do not need to lose a large amount of weight to help your body metabolically. A weight reduction of 5 pounds is definitely helpful. However, I am sure many of you feel that you can lose more. Simply take another month on the **Weight Reduction Mode** and work on another 5 pounds.

I have done a study on my patients using my daily weighing program over the past year with tremendous success. So far I have over 140 patients using the Chang Method, and 93% succeeded in losing an average of 10 pounds. In fact, my program is so successful that it is very unusual to have anyone gain weight on it.

Most of the so-called "failures" are people who

did not have any weight changes. One of my patients who gained weight on this program was a woman who started weighing herself daily for two months and gained 1 pound. It turned out that she also started exercising during those two months by rowing with the women's rowing team for one and a half hours, three times a week. Even though I list her in my study as a "failure," I feel that she was actually a success because she probably gained many pounds of muscle and lost as many pounds of fat.

Another instance of weight gain on my program involved a patient who gained 4 pounds, from 210 pounds to 214 pounds over three months, while weighing himself every day. I was so puzzled by this that I asked him if he tested the accuracy of his scale by stepping on it three times in a row. He replied that, indeed, he did and he got three different readings: 213, 220 and 215. I advised him to get a new scale and start all over again.

There is also a national study involving more than 3,000 patients over a six-year period that supports my daily weighing program. To read more about my study and the national study, please refer to the Appendix.

There are several advantages to my daily weighing method. One is that it is compatible with all of the dieting programs around. Another is that my program is absolutely free. The only thing it may cost you is the price of a good scale. And finally, it is entirely safe and effective.

There are two important differences between my weight loss program and most of the other dieting programs you hear about.

First, the key to my program is weighing yourself every day. To my knowledge, none of the other dieting programs recommends this. In fact, many of these programs actually discourage people from daily weighing. This is analogous to asking diabetics to control their disease without checking their blood sugar regularly, or to asking business people to succeed without checking their cash registers every day. Weight control is no different. To be successful in controlling your weight, you must weigh yourself every day.

Let me share with you what my patients say about daily weighing. Sarah, who was initially doubtful, wrote: "I was skeptical when Dr. Chang introduced the daily weighing program. I felt it was not necessary, especially since all of the diet programs I had been to in the past said weigh once a week. But I found that weighing myself daily gives me much more motivation to stick to my diabetic weight loss regimen...This plan has really worked for me."

Gina, who was warned by others not to weigh herself daily, wrote: "The weight got away from me while others encouraged me to, 'Oh, only weigh once a week. Why do that misery to yourself everyday?' Well, forget everyone else, now I weigh in every day and I have a handle on my own weight and life, and it's not misery. It's like it's a game. I now adjust my food intake accordingly. Thank you, Dr. Chang, for introducing me to this way of thinking. I'm hooked for life."

Hillary, who had previously failed on every diet she had tried, wrote: "Dr. Chang said the key to losing weight was weighing every day. My immediate reaction was what does this healthy slim doctor know about weight loss? He tells me to do something that was against all of the diet programs that I had ever been on. And let me tell you, I have been on almost every imaginable diet. When I left I thought about what he had said and decided I would try it. I have lost over 20 pounds and it has been gradual and with little effort. I cut way back on meats and decreased fats and sugar. I do not count calories or points or how many of what foods I have consumed in a day. I just weigh every morning and it keeps me focused all day. I have recommended this to many of my friends."

Nancy, who had succeeded in maintaining an over 80 pound weight loss, wrote: "For 30 years I had been told repeatedly not to get on the scale more that once a week and not to obsess with my daily weight fluctuations. This advice, no matter how well intentioned, was just plain wrong."

Weighing daily makes my patients feel in control of their weight. Emmet wrote: "Daily weighing has helped me keep my weight in check, especially during the holidays. I now feel in control of my weight and am confident that I can meet my weight loss goals."

Rebecca wrote: "I'm back, 30 pounds lighter,

better fit than I've been in years—just in time to greet my 50th birthday this year. I'm still exercising and following Weight Watcher's awareness of daily food intake—minimum and maximum. And I'm not afraid of daily weigh-ins. They simply keep me on track and help me catch myself before my weight gets out of hand again. I enjoy being accountable and in control, not to mention just feeling awfully good in my clothes!"

Nora wrote: "I have tried many forms of weight reduction over the years but have never felt as 'in control' and inspired as I do following Dr. Chang's plan. Knowing that I will be stepping on that scale in the morning makes me very aware of exactly what I am eating."

The second striking difference between my weight loss program and all of the other dieting programs is my emphasis on the **Weight Maintenance Mode** and starting out with this mode for a period of time before going on the **Weight Reduction Mode**. Most other programs either do not have the very important weight maintenance component, or if they do, they put it after the weight reduction phase and do not emphasize its importance. The problem with this approach is that to start off with the more difficult weight reduction phase can be very discouraging, causing some to drop out. The ones who are able to achieve weight loss often feel so deprived that they go right back to their previous life style and end up gaining all the weight back before they know it, especially since they don't weigh themselves daily. There is little positive reinforcement and the dieters frequently feel like failures.

My program is unique in that it starts off with the **Weight Maintenance Mode**, which is easier to accomplish. Success here is defined as maintaining your weight. You do not need to lose weight to feel successful. All you need to do is not gain weight. Most of you can achieve this. When you are ready, you will enter the **Weight Reduction Mode** feeling very positive and successful. The weight reduction goal you will set is realistic and practical, so that it is very achievable. Finally, after you achieve the weight reduction, you will go right back to the now very familiar **Weight Maintenance Mode** and you will achieve permanent weight loss. It is easy to see why over 90% of my patients succeed in losing weight using the Chang Method.

● To Summarize
- Be sure to have a reliable scale and weigh yourself once a day at the same time.
- Start with the **Weight Maintenance Mode**. Keep from gaining any weight by acting on any weight gain you detect from one day to the next. Be patient, because it may take a few days to drop the pound or two that you gained. You should feel like a success if you are able to maintain your weight.
- After a period of successful weight maintenance, start on the **Weight Reduction Mode**. Set a realistic goal,

such as losing 5 pounds over a month. Think of it as a temporary sacrifice for a healthier future life.

- Once you achieve this goal, get right back on the **Weight Maintenance Mode** so that you will never gain the weight back.
- Repeat this small weight loss as many times as you need to reach your final weight loss goal. You may have set this at 20 pounds. This will require you to repeat your weight loss month three more times.
- Just get back on the **Weight Maintenance Mode** when you feel that you have reached your final goal weight.

Besides weight maintenance, of course, true weight loss depends on the other two factors: diet and exercise. I will cover these in Chapters 3 and 4. It is, however, important at first to learn how to maintain your weight and to practice this for a period of time.

It is very important that you follow the above steps exactly in order to succeed in using the Chang Method. For that reason, I will repeat this summary at the end of the book.

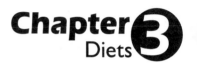

Chapter 3
Diets

I feel that any discussion of diets is redundant because there has been so much written about them. To add further to the confusion, many of these diets contradict each other. Today, Americans spend over $30 billion annually on diet products. Manufacturers of food, appliances, pills, and owners of clubs, clinics, and salons constantly hype that they are selling the solution everyone has been waiting for. In addition, every year publishers give us a crop of brand new diets to try.

The fact that there are so many diets and more keep popping up every year means only one thing—none of them works perfectly. If they did, we would have exactly one recommended diet. Also, the rate of obesity would be going down instead of going up. Americans would be winning instead of losing the battle of the bulge.

• The Three Major Diet Types

There are three major types of diets based on

the calories derived from fat, carbohydrates (CHO) and protein. One of them is the high-fat, low-carbohydrate, high-protein diet represented by the Atkins diet. The second is the low-fat or very low-fat diet. The third is the moderate-fat, high-carbohydrate, moderate-protein diet. Let's look at each one briefly.

● The High-Fat, Low-Carbohydrate Diet

The Atkins diet is the best known high-protein, high-fat, and very-low-carbohydrate diet. It emphasizes meat, cheese and eggs, while discouraging foods such as bread, pasta, fruit, and sugar.

The Atkins diet basically says you can eat as much fat and protein as you want, but you must restrict the carbohydrates to a very low level, starting at 20 grams or less per day. It says that calories don't matter, that carbohydrates make the body more apt to gain weight regardless of calories, and that going on this diet will make you lose weight regardless of calorie intake. Since there are no limits on the quantities of foods permitted on the diet, you don't have to be hungry between meals.

Generally, dieters on high-fat, low-carbohydrate diets, such as the Atkins diet, lose weight at a faster rate initially than those on the other diets. However, this is only a temporary phenomenon, lasting just a short time due to a greater loss of body water than body fat. Ultimately, the rate of weight loss equalizes between the different diets. This is because, as reliable studies show, calories *do* matter and people lose weight when they consume fewer calories, regardless of the fat or carbohydrate contents of the diets.

Although these high-fat, low-carbohydrate diets claim that people can eat unlimited calories and lose weight, studies have shown that, in actuality, people on these diets consume fewer calories. Of course, consuming fewer calories is why they lose weight. I have talked with people who say that this diet worked for them. However, it is difficult for many people to stay on such a restricted diet for a prolonged period of time. Under the Chang Method, you can certainly use the high-fat, low-carbohydrate diet during the **Weight Reduction Mode** as long as you resume the **Weight Maintenance Mode** to keep the weight off forever.

High-fat, low-carbohydrate diets can have negative effects on your body. They result in ketosis, which can cause an increase in uric acid concentrations in the blood. High uric acid may cause kidney stones and arthritis. In addition, these high-fat diets lower LDL cholesterol (the bad cholesterol) less than the low-fat diets do. They also tend to be low in certain vitamins and minerals as well as dietary fiber, and require vitamin supplements to make up for their many nutritional deficiencies. Finally, increase in red meat consumption may increase the risk of a number of different cancers, including breast, colon, prostate, kidney, and pancreas.

● The Low-Fat Diet or Very-Low-Fat Diet

The most well known of these are the Pritikin and Ornish programs. The Pritikin diet is almost completely vegetarian and encourages the consumption of large amounts of whole grains and vegetables. It is high in fiber, low in cholesterol, and extremely low in saturated fat and total fat. On the low-fat diet, fat consumption is restricted to 11% to 19% per day. The very-low-fat diet restricts fats to less than 10%. Individuals following the diet are encouraged to eat six or seven meals each day and are not required to restrict portion sizes. The diet excludes nearly all processed grains and sources of animal protein. These diets stress very high carbohydrate and moderate protein consumption.

Originally, these low-fat diet programs were created to reverse and prevent heart disease. They also resulted in weight loss. Because Americans are increasingly overweight and desperate to lose that weight, the focus of these diets has changed from treating heart disease as the main goal to weight loss.

These low-fat diets generally work on a short-term basis. However, because they are so restrictive they are difficult to stay on for more than a few months. For some people, these diets are appropriate and work well with the Chang Method. Because meat and fat intake is severely restricted, it is important to supplement with additional vitamins such as vitamin E and zinc.

● **The Moderate-Fat, High-Carbohydrate Diet**

The USDA Food Guide Pyramid and the Weight Watchers program exemplify this diet. At the top of the pyramid are fats, oils and sweets...next come the milk, yogurt and cheese group... the meat, poultry, fish, dry beans, eggs and nuts group...the vegetable group, fruit group... and the bread, cereal, rice and pasta group. This diet is 20% to 30% fat, high in carbohydrates and moderate in protein.

To use the Pyramid, start with plenty of breads, cereals, rice, pasta, vegetables, and fruits. Add two to three servings from the milk group and two to three servings from the meat group. Remember to go easy on fats, oils, and sweets, the foods in the small tip of the Pyramid. The Weight Watchers program assigns points to each type of food. Dieters are allowed to pick anything they want, up to the assigned number of points.

Weight Watchers is the diet that I prefer for my patients because it is nutritionally balanced, better lowers LDL cholesterol (the bad cholesterol), and offers more food choices than the other diets. It's very flexible and can easily be followed. People don't feel as deprived and, as a result, can stay on it much longer than on the other diets. This is very important because the goal is to stay on this diet long term. In fact, the ideal would be to stay on it forever.

Let me explain my recommended diet a

little further. I prefer the fat consumed to include mostly monounsaturated or polyunsaturated fats. Monounsaturated fats include olive oil, canola oil, and nuts. Polyunsaturated fats include the omega-3 fatty acids, which are found in fish and vegetables. It is important to avoid saturated fats, which are found in red meat, butter, cheese and milk. It is especially important to avoid a type of fat called trans-fatty acids. Some examples of foods in which these are found are margarine, shortening and fried fast foods.

Whole grains, fruits and vegetables are your best sources of carbohydrates. In our modern grocery stores, there is a wide variety of healthy food choices available.

All of these diets work as long as you reduce the total caloric intake. You can lose weight on any diet that lowers calories.   However, you are not going to be able to keep it off if you are always hungry and dissatisfied with a limited choice of foods. What we are seeking is a permanent change that you can happily live with, not a quick fix that will end up being just one more failure.

My approach to counseling my patients on the moderate-fat diet differs somewhat from the usual approach recommended by organizations such as the National Institutes of Health, the National Cholesterol Education Program or by most dietitians. The standard, very complicated approach is to recommend something like the following: restricting the daily intake of saturated fat to less than 10% of total calories, and the daily intake of total fat to less than 30% of total calories. To carry this out, a person has to figure out the total calories, which is usually a fairly large number (e.g., 1,500 to 2,000), take 8% to 10% of this, and divide this by 9 (since there are 9 calories per gram of fat), to find out what the number of grams of saturated fat should be. Then this process is repeated for the total fat. Now the individual is ready to read the labels on everything he eats, adding up the saturated fat and the total fat separately to be sure he does not exceed the quota.

I contend that it takes a highly motivated person who is very good in math, such as a rocket scientist carrying a calculator at all times, to carry out the above diet recommendations.

I use a much simpler approach for my patients. I recommend to them only one number: the number of grams of total fat per day. This usually ranges between 40 grams to 80 grams per day, depending on their weight. I then give them a one-page list of the fat contents of common food items that they can tape to their refrigerator door for easy reference. I believe that this approach is easy to follow and many of my patients have lost weight as well as lowered their cholesterol using it.

Let me illustrate how this diet lowers cholesterol with examples using two of my patients. Mark was a 53-year-old gentleman with high cholesterol whom I put on a diet of 40 grams of fat per day. His initial total cholesterol was 252. His LDL (the bad cholesterol) was 182. These numbers were very high. After three months on the diet with no medications, his total cholesterol dropped an amazing 68 points or 27%. His LDL dropped an even more amazing 51 points or 28%. Now Mark's cholesterol is completely normal and his chance of developing heart disease is greatly reduced.

The second example is a 42-year-old gentleman named Jim, who had a very high total cholesterol of 270. He had an LDL of 172. I also put him on a diet of 40 grams of fat per day. In four months his total cholesterol dropped 37 points or 14%. Jim's LDL dropped an incredible 42 points or 24%. Again, without medicine, he was able to greatly reduce his risk of developing heart disease. These are but two of many examples of how my patients have benefitted greatly from my program.

Donna, who was very happy with the Chang Method, wrote: "Several months ago I met my new doctor, Dr. Chang. I was a little apprehensive since I had packed on quite a few pounds over the last few years and my blood pressure was moderately high. Dr. Chang provided me with some clear information on achieving and maintaining weight loss. The doctor gave me three simple guidelines to follow:

- Eat no more than 40 grams of fat a day.
- Exercise for twenty minutes at least five to seven days a week.
- Weigh myself at the same time every day.

By applying Dr. Chang's medical regimen, I had significant decreases: blood pressure, weight, cholesterol, and bad cholesterol (LDL). I definitely feel a lot better. I have more energy and more confidence in myself to continue my new lifestyle changes. Thank you very much, Dr. Chang."

And finally, I have some helpful hints for you on how to reduce the amount of calories you consume. As the stomach fills up, it sends a signal to the brain to tell it that it is no longer hungry and to stop eating. This may take a little while, so it is important to use techniques to enable this signal to get to the brain before you overeat. Some techniques are to eat slowly and drink a non-creamy soup or water at the beginning of the meal. Also, sit down while you eat, eat regular meals, and don't skip meals so that you get overly hungry. In addition, most of us are conditioned to eat everything on the plate, so when going to restaurants get a doggy bag before the meal and put a portion of the food in it before you start eating to avoid overeating. As a general rule, avoid fast foods. If you must have fast food, try to avoid the fried foods. If you just can't resist them, do not "supersize!"

These recommendations will help you lose weight. Additionally, use the daily weighing method described in Chapter 2 to monitor your weight loss progress. If you do this, you are sure to succeed in losing weight and keeping it off forever.

Chapter 4
Exercise and Weight Loss

Exercise is an important factor in fighting obesity. It is virtually impossible to lose weight and maintain the weight reduction without it. Exercise is the important third leg of the Chang Method. However, to be successful, an exercise program has to be practical and simple to follow.

I always recommend that my patients exercise a minimum of twenty minutes a day using an aerobic-type exercise. The definition of aerobic exercise is continuous exercise using large muscles. Some examples of aerobic exercise are brisk walking, cycling, using a treadmill or stationary bike, and swimming. Brisk walking is actually the most widely accepted and well-proven effective exercise. However, I recommend buying exercise equipment as an alternative, if feasible, since the weather and other factors may make it impossible to walk outside on a daily basis. Some of the exercise equipment includes stationary bicycles, treadmills, stair steppers/climbers, ski machines, and jogging trampolines.

Which equipment you purchase is entirely up to you. However, I am including a breakdown here to help you get started.

● Aerobic Fitness Equipment

- **Stationary bicycles** work the legs through the pedaling motion of a bicycle. Some models are used sitting upright, others recumbent (seated leaning back).
- **Treadmills** let you walk or run at varying speeds. Some models simulate inclines of various degrees, and many incorporate timers.
- **Stair steppers/climbers** duplicate the motion of climbing up a flight of stairs. Some add upper body exercise by simulating a pull-up climbing motion with the arms.
- **Ski machines** simulate the motion of cross-country skiing and exercise the legs and arms simultaneously.
- **Elliptical trainers** are a cross between a ski machine and a stair stepper, and exercise your legs and feet in a circular, up-and-down motion.
- **Rowing machines** work the back, arms and legs.
- **Aerobic riders** exercise the arms and legs simultaneously through a push/pull motion.

To avoid purchasing the wrong equipment, you need to give this some thought. Here are some of the questions to ask yourself. What activities do I enjoy most? Which don't I like? If you avoid taking stairs at all costs, you probably will not like working out on a stair climber/stepper, decreasing the chances you will use it regularly. If you love to take brisk walks, a treadmill will give you a similar experience any time, day or night, in any type of weather. The more you enjoy the activity your equipment provides, the more often you will use it.

How much do you have to spend? Decide on a budget. If you love that fancy, programmable $2,500 stair climber at the gym, the $199 blue-light special will probably prove to be a huge disappointment—but a basic, quality $600 to $800 model might work well. A good strategy is to spend most of your budget on one solid aerobic training piece, say a high-quality treadmill, then build around it with inexpensive strength training equipment such as tubing and dumbbells.

What features do you really need? Decide on features and functions: from televised displays to digital readouts, much of today's equipment incorporates an amazing amount of high technology. However, these "bells and whistles" often come at a price. Ask yourself if timers, heart rate monitors, calories-burned displays and the like will motivate you. If so, and you can afford them, great. If not, rest assured that a basic, good-quality piece will provide just as effective a workout. And you can often duplicate many features by using kitchen timers, keeping an exercise log with handwritten entries, and even learning how to take your own pulse.

What else do you need? Other considerations include a reading rack, ease of adjusting variables such as tension, resistance and seat height, water bottle holders, and whether it folds up.

Ask questions! Ask about warranties, return policies, satisfaction guarantees, frequency and cost of repairs. In some cases, a reputable dealer will let you try out your new equipment at home for a specified time period, say thirty days, and allow you to return it for a full refund or merchandise credit if you are not satisfied. The dealer may take care of pick-up, delivery and set-up.

● My Experience

Let me share with you my exercise preference. I exercise at least twenty minutes a day. I do this mainly for stress reduction and to keep my weight down. I must confess that I hate aerobic exercise of any kind. I used to enjoy playing tennis but, as I wrote earlier, I quit due to a shoulder injury about ten years ago.

So I had to find some kind of aerobic exercise. Unfortunately, I hate walking or jogging. I have difficulty using the treadmill due to an inner ear problem. I cannot stand exercising sitting down, such as cycling. I find the ski machines tearfully boring. The only equipment I found which I could tolerate was the StairMaster. However, that cost over $2,000. I saw an ad for a stair stepper for only $200, which I thought was based on a similar mechanism as the StairMaster. I rushed out and bought this machine.

Unfortunately, I only used the stepper twice and never used it again. I ended up giving it away and bought the more expensive StairMaster. I have been using it almost daily now for nearly ten years. The reason I like the StairMaster is that I can read while exercising. I also have a TV in front of it, which helps a great deal to take my mind off the tedium of daily exercise. My advice to my patients as to which exercise equipment to get is to be sure to try it out for a few times before purchasing it. Also, it is always a good idea to have some distraction such as a radio, TV, or reading to combat the monotony of daily exercise.

A young physician friend of mine came to me as a patient five years ago. He was healthy and took fairly good care of himself. He did not smoke cigarettes or drink alcohol excessively. His blood pressure and cholesterol were both normal. The only thing missing was regular exercise, and as a result he had gained some weight. After my discussion about the importance of daily exercise with him, he decided to get a StairMaster also. In fact, I had him call my wife at home to get the telephone number to order the machine. He has been using it religiously. He lost 20 pounds after a few months and has kept his weight down ever since.

● What About Heart Rate?

Some experts feel that in order to benefit the

heart, it is necessary to achieve and maintain a certain heart rate while exercising. I don't subscribe to this belief because I think it is too cumbersome for many people and may discourage them from exercising. It is important to keep it simple. Just remember to exercise every day for at least twenty minutes.

It is also important to avoid overexertion. You can recognize that you are overexerting when you can't carry on a conversation while exercising due to shortness of breath. This indicates that the body is no longer in an aerobic state but rather in anaerobic state where there is insufficient oxygen.

● Other Benefits of Exercise

Exercise, of course, provides an essential weight-loss tool, but it also has many other health benefits. First, just two and a half hours of exercise a week drastically lowers the incidence of diabetes. We have known for a long time that exercise helps people with diabetes to control their disease better, often enabling them to require fewer medications such as diabetes pills or insulin shots. A recent study involving several thousand obese patients who were prone to have diabetes showed that two and a half hours of exercise a week, such a brisk walking, plus a 5% weight loss, lowered the incidence of diabetes by a whopping 58%! I will elaborate on this very exciting study in more detail in the next chapter.

Moderate exercise has many other major health

benefits. Various studies of the effects of exercise on both men and women show reduction in the risk of heart disease by up to 40%. This also applies to the risk of stroke. Exercise helps to lower high blood pressure. It increases the amount of HDL, or good cholesterol, which helps to reduce cardiovascular disease. It reduces the risk of osteoporosis, which is the most common cause of hip fractures. Some studies even suggest that exercise can lower the risk of certain cancers, such as colon cancer.

Exercise helps to reduce stress. Under stress, the body secretes stress hormones such as adrenaline, which is also known as the "Fight or Flight" hormone. Adrenaline was a very important hormone for prehistoric man when facing a wild animal because it enabled him to run into his cave to hide or to fight back.

Fortunately for modern man, we have very little need for this reaction. Nevertheless, most of us face stress every day whether it is from work or from home. Adrenaline is secreted daily but is not used up. Rather, it keeps accumulating and causes muscle contractions throughout the body, often creating tension headaches due to contraction of the muscles of the scalp. Similar muscle spasms, caused by stress, create neck pain, backache and chest wall pain.

Our intestines are also lined with muscles, and contraction of these muscles causes spastic colon or irritable bowel syndrome. The symptoms of irritable bowel syndrome include abdominal pain, nausea, bloating, constipation and diarrhea.

Blood pressure can go up due to contraction of the smooth muscles in the arterial walls. Adrenaline can also increase acid secretion in the stomach, which can result in heartburn and peptic ulcers. Other detrimental effects of built-up adrenaline include anxiety, insomnia and depression.

For good health, it is necessary to cleanse the body of the built-up adrenaline. This can be achieved by using up the adrenaline. Exercising is the way to use up the adrenaline. That is why it is so important to exercise on a daily basis.

Finally, there is a study on long-term successful weight reduction called the National Weight Control Registry. This is the only long-term study of weight loss to date (most studies range from a few weeks to a few months). The subjects in this study were able to maintain an amazing 60 pounds of weight loss over an incredibly long length of time—six years. The study found that three behaviors accounted for the tremendous success of this group. First, subjects ate a low-fat, low-calorie diet. Second, they monitored their weight regularly. Third, they exercised an average of sixty to ninety minutes a day. The most common form of exercise was brisk walking (see Appendix).

This chapter illustrates the tremendous importance of regular exercise. Exercise is essential to helping you lose weight and maintain your weight loss. It can also help you prevent many future health problems, both physical and mental. It is relatively inexpensive to do and can help you avoid medications that can have many adverse side effects. I strongly urge you to get in the habit of doing at least twenty minutes of aerobic exercise every day. This is one habit that will benefit you for the rest of your life.

Chapter 5
Diabetes Prevention

Diabetes is a disease with profound adverse effects on longevity as well as on the quality of life. It is obvious that we can save people from a lot of suffering if we can prevent diabetes.

Approximately 8% of adult Americans today have diabetes, a condition marked by high levels of sugar in the blood. The vast majority (90% to 95%) has what is known as type 2 diabetes. This type of diabetes typically occurs in middle life or later.

People with type 2 diabetes are not able to make enough insulin or they simply do not respond normally to the insulin that their bodies make. This inability to make enough insulin or to properly utilize it causes sugar (glucose) to build up in the blood. Over time, high levels of sugar in the blood can lead to serious medical problems, including kidney disease, eye disease, heart disease, strokes and poor circulation.

Unfortunately, it is not easy to control diabetes and bring the blood sugar level into a normal range. Furthermore, even optimal control of diabetes does not completely eliminate its devastating complications. Therefore, it is much better to prevent the adverse consequences of diabetes by preventing the disease.

A recent study reported in the *New England Journal of Medicine* examined the effectiveness of weight loss and exercise in preventing diabetes. It was also one of the few times that anyone looked at the effectiveness of a diabetes medication in the prevention of diabetes.

● The *New England Journal of Medicine* Study

The February 2002 issue of the *New England Journal of Medicine* discussed a program that effectively lowers the risk of diabetes. This study involved over 3,000 overweight people whose blood sugars were close to diabetes range. These were individuals who were at extremely high risk of developing diabetes. The design of the study was to see if it was possible to prevent diabetes in this group. The participants were randomly assigned to three groups. The first group was treated with intensive lifestyle intervention. The second group received standard lifestyle intervention plus a placebo. The third group was given standard lifestyle intervention plus metformin, a diabetes medication normally given to patients who already have developed diabetes. They were followed for three years.

Intensive lifestyle intervention included a healthy low-fat, low-calorie diet and an exercise program consisting of at least two and a half hours per week of physical activity of moderate intensity such as brisk walking (covered in Chapter 4). These participants also went through a sixteen-lesson curriculum covering diet, exercise, and behavior modification taught by counselors during the first twenty-four weeks after enrollment.

The standard lifestyle intervention consisted of only one annual thirty-minute individual session that emphasized the importance of a healthy lifestyle. Participants were encouraged to follow the Food Guide Pyramid, to reduce their weight and to increase their physical activity.

People on the intensive lifestyle intervention lost an average of 7% of their body weight, or approximately 15 pounds, during the first year. They sustained a 5% reduction of their body weight for the remaining two years of the study. These lifestyle changes resulted in a marked reduction in the risk of diabetes.

At the end of three years, the rate of development of diabetes in the placebo group was 11%, in the metformin group it was 8%, and in the intensive lifestyle intervention group it was only 5%. Another way to look at this is that intensive lifestyle intervention reduced the risk of diabetes by 58% compared to placebo. Intensive lifestyle intervention, then, dramatically lowers the rate of diabetes.

● Prescription Drug Use

As I mentioned above, this was one of the few studies that tested the effectiveness of an oral hypoglycemic agent (a medication that lowers blood sugar) in the prevention of diabetes. Traditionally we only use these medications on people who have developed diabetes. The medication used in this study was metformin, a relatively newer class of oral diabetes medication. The older class of oral diabetes medication is known as sulfonylureas. Some examples of these are glyburide, glipizide, and tolbutamide. These sulfonylureas act primarily by increasing the secretion of insulin from the pancreas, which helps to lower the blood sugar.

Metformin, on the other hand, acts mainly by making the liver and muscles more sensitive to the effects of insulin, so that it takes less insulin to lower blood sugar. Additionally, metformin decreases the amount of sugar the liver makes. The overall effect is that metformin lowers blood sugar and conserves insulin. It does not lower blood sugar too much if the patient forgets to eat, as the sulfonylureas tend to do. Finally, a beneficial side effect of metformin is that it may cause some weight loss, which is good for diabetics. The *New England Journal of Medicine* study showed that metformin, when given to people who were prone to have diabetes, did indeed help to reduce the incidence of the disease.

● The Implications of the Study

As you can see, exercise, weight loss, and

metformin reduced the incidence of diabetes. This means essentially that by building a healthy lifestyle, you can decrease your chance of getting diabetes and still do the things you enjoy most—such as traveling, socializing, and having fun. A healthy lifestyle includes exercising and keeping your weight under control.

To have an effect, you need to maintain a weight reduction of 5% and exercise two and a half hours a week. This shouldn't be too difficult to do since my patients, using the Chang Method discussed in Chapter 2, lost almost 5% of their weight in six months. See Chapters 2 and 4 for an effective weight loss and exercise program.

Changing to a healthy lifestyle dramatically lowers the risk of diabetes. Just imagine—if the high-risk people combined this relatively easy-to-achieve intensive lifestyle intervention with metformin, they could potentially drop their chance of becoming diabetics to as low as one or two percent.

One of my patients, William, was able to achieve a healthier lifestyle using my daily weighing program and wrote: "I have diabetes and high blood pressure but have been able to avoid medication for the diabetes through exercise and weight control. The weight control is accomplished by weighing myself about five times a week on the average. Daily weighing lets me know if I ate too much in one day. If I have put on weight, then I have to watch what I eat closely for a few days until the weight goes down. This works well for maintaining my blood sugar readings and I am able to understand why my blood pressure readings are what they are. I believe the daily weighing helps me maintain a healthier lifestyle and makes me feel better."

In conclusion, to avoid getting diabetes it is important to get on an effective exercise/weight loss program. The results could be dramatic.

Chapter 6
How To Stop Smoking

Weight loss benefits most of us. It is especially helpful for smokers who are trying to quit. This is because one of the impediments to quitting smoking is the weight gain associated with it. This is not a myth, it is real. It is not unusual for my patients to report a 10 to 20 pound weight gain after quitting cigarettes. Following the weight maintenance program described in Chapter 2 can prevent this.

Now let me give you some useful hints to motivate you. Most people know that smoking is bad for the lungs, causing conditions such as emphysema and lung cancer. Some of you may not know that smoking increases the incidence of many other cancers such as colon and bladder cancer. In fact, some urologists claim that nearly 100% of those with bladder cancer have smoked cigarettes. Also, smoking is bad for the heart, increasing the risk of heart attacks. It is bad for the circulation, causing strokes, leg pain and in severe cases, loss of limbs.

Stopping smoking is not easy. In my medical career I have seen a number of people quit. A small number quit after I counseled them. Most of the rest quit after a catastrophic event, most commonly either a stroke or heart attack. Unfortunately, not everyone survives a stroke or heart attack. But even if a person survives these catastrophic events, he or she is usually permanently damaged.

Although I have never smoked cigarettes, I can understand how difficult it is to quit. I would like to illustrate this using my patient whom I will call Virginia.

Virginia had circulatory problems due to her cigarette smoking. She developed Transient Ischemic Attacks (TIA's), which are sometimes known as mini-strokes. TIA's are typically manifested by stroke-like symptoms, such as weakness on one side of the body or loss of speech, which go away after less than twenty-four hours. Many people who have had TIA's later suffer major strokes. Virginia would experience symptoms of weakness on the left side of her body lasting for about an hour. The workup of her TIA's revealed a nearly completely clogged carotid artery on the right side of her neck. This artery supplies blood to the brain. I recommended that she undergo an operation to open up the clogged carotid artery to prevent a completed or permanent stroke.

I also strongly recommended that she stop smoking

to prevent circulation problems elsewhere. Virginia underwent a successful carotid surgery but was unable to stop smoking. Later, she developed similar problems involving the right side of her body along with a speech problem due to occlusion of her left carotid artery. She fortunately had another successful operation on her left carotid artery, which again prevented her from having permanent neurological problems. Unfortunately, she was still unable to stop smoking.

Next, Virginia began having pain in her left foot at rest due to poor circulation. This progressed to her toes turning black or gangrenous, requiring amputation. She continued to smoke. Later, gangrene spread to her left leg and she ended up having a below-the-knee amputation. None of this, however, caused her to stop smoking, despite my repeated warnings that her life and health depended on it. Then her right leg developed problems, ending in amputation below the knee. At this point, Virginia had undergone two major surgeries of her carotid arteries and had lost both of her legs to smoking, but she still couldn't stop. This illustrated to me how addictive cigarettes could be. I figured that Virginia would never stop smoking. A year later, Virginia had a heart attack and guess what—that gave her the will power to stop. Unfortunately, she died not too long afterwards.

I have since related Virginia's tragic story to some of my patients who smoke. I also tell them that most people stop smoking following catastrophic events such as heart attacks and strokes. It is the exceptional people who can stop before these events occur. Interestingly enough, I have been able to help a few, the exceptional ones, to give up this dangerous habit.

● How to Stop Smoking

Studies show that the best approach to quitting is to use some kind of nicotine substitute, such as the nicotine patch, along with enrolling in a behavioral modification program. If this fails, it is reasonable to try the prescription medicine, Zyban, which is an antidepressant medication. Check with your physician.

To be successful quitting, you must want to stop. Without a strong commitment on your part, it just won't happen. One of the big fears of most smokers is that if they quit, they will gain weight. This fear is justified. However, by using the maintenance program described in Chapter 2, you will find it possible to keep weight gain to a minimum.

Chapter 7
High Blood Pressure

One of the many benefits of weight reduction is the lowering of high blood pressure. High blood pressure, also known as hypertension, is defined as blood pressure over 140/90. It is a very common medical problem, affecting nearly half of our adult population. It is associated with increased incidence of strokes, heart attacks, heart failure (or fluid in the lungs), and kidney failure. The higher the blood pressure, the higher the chance of these complications. Lowering blood pressure reduces complications. One scary thing about high blood pressure is that it does not have any symptoms. A person with very high blood pressure may feel perfectly fine until he or she has a stroke or heart attack. This is why hypertension is often called the silent killer. It is important for all of us to have our blood pressure checked at least once a year, and to have high blood pressure treated.

To treat hypertension, it is important to try lifestyle adjustment first. Lifestyle adjustment involves a low-salt diet, exercise, and weight loss for those who are overweight. A low-salt diet means not adding salt to your food and avoiding foods with a lot of salt. Most people know that foods such as pickles, potato chips and soy sauce are loaded with salt. I also tell my patients to avoid canned soup, canned vegetables and other canned foods. I had a patient whose blood pressure was difficult to control. He carefully watched his salt intake. However, upon closer questioning, I found that he ate out a lot and always ordered soup. I told him that soup served in restaurants usually contains a lot of salt. Since he stopped ordering soup, his blood pressure has come down to normal.

To control hypertension, I recommend twenty minutes of aerobic type of exercise a day. Permanent weight loss is important in both the prevention and the treatment of hypertension for those who are overweight. There are many examples of this with my patients. One patient in her early 60s had an elevated blood pressure of 146/92. I instructed her to go on my daily weighing program and to exercise regularly. She returned in five months having lost 6 pounds. She also exercised by walking twenty minutes a day. Her blood pressure dropped to 138/80 without any medications. Another patient lost a remarkable 42 pounds of weight in three months following my program and dropped his blood pressure from 154/86 to 136/80. If the blood pressure is still high despite lifestyle adjustment, medication will be needed.

When I was in medical school over thirty years ago, there were only a handful of drugs available to treat hypertension. These included diuretics (water pills) and three or four other drugs. How simple it was to practice medicine then! Since then there has been a number of new classes of blood pressure medications, such as beta-blockers, calcium channel blockers, angiotensin-converting enzyme (ACE) inhibitors, angiotensin-receptor blockers and more. However, most of these newer medications are expensive, sometimes costing hundreds of dollars a month. Health insurance often does not cover their cost, leaving many patients, especially seniors on a fixed income, in a bind.

Doctors began prescribing these newer, more expensive medications because studies seemed to show that they were far more effective than older treatments such as diuretics. As a result, from 1982 to 1992 there was a decline in the use of diuretics from 56% to 27%. That was a big factor in the huge increase in hypertension treatment cost. It is estimated that Americans spend $15.5 billion on blood pressure medications each year in this country.

Well, there is good news for people with hypertension who are on a limited budget. The National Institutes of Health (NIH) just completed a study called the

Antihypertensive and Lipid-Lowering Treatment to Prevent Heart Attack Trial (ALLHAT). This study, conducted from February 1994 through March 2002, involved over 30,000 patients. The object of the study was to see if treating hypertension with two of the newer types of medications, namely an ACE inhibitor and a calcium channel blocker, works better than using a diuretic. The study compared these three types of medications in terms of their effectiveness in lowering blood pressure as well as their ability to lower heart disease and strokes.

Guess what? The conclusion of ALLHAT was that the diuretics were just as effective in lowering blood pressure and preventing heart disease and strokes as the ACE inhibitor and the calcium channel blocker. Actually, in some of the categories the diuretic was superior. Indeed, the cheapest was the best.

I can attest to the effectiveness of diuretics in controlling high blood pressure in many of my patients. This is especially true in people over the age of 60. I recently saw a patient in his late 60s with an elevated blood pressure of 158/96. I put him on my daily weighing program and a diuretic. He returned to see me in two months and had achieved a weight loss of 17 pounds. His blood pressure had dropped to normal at 120/70. He is one of many of my patients who have successfully controlled their blood pressures through weight loss and diuretics.

This is good news for hypertensive patients

because diuretics are much less expensive, costing on an average about one-fifth as much as the other classes of hypertensive medications. This will make treating hypertension much more affordable for many people without compromising the quality of care.

Remember, however, that it is always better to prevent a disease than to treat it. Hypertension is no exception. It is well established that proper diet, exercise, and weight loss can prevent hypertension and avoid the need for medication for many people. Using the Chang Method of weight loss can benefit your health in many ways, including preventing high blood pressure.

Chapter 8
Take Care of Your Joints

Exercise plays an extremely important role both in weight loss and in maintenance of weight loss. It is essential to take care of your joints so that you can avoid injuries and continue to exercise as long as possible. I would like to share with you my approach to taking care of two orthopedic problems that frequently interfere with people's ability to exercise: knee pain and back pain.

Many people think that orthopedic problems such as osteoarthritis (degenerative joint disease) are permanent, and that the only definitive treatment is surgery. It is true that once osteoarthritis is present, it will always be there. However, it is possible to reduce the symptoms of pain as well as improve the function of the joints by following the appropriate treatment. My recommendations on how to treat osteoarthritis are to avoid stress to the joint involved, strengthen the muscles that move the joint, and take a nonsteroidal anti-inflammatory medication, such as ibuprofen and naproxen, if there are no contraindications. Physical therapy can also be very helpful.

Let me give you an example. My father-in-law, Vernon, who is currently 91, was having a lot of problems with his knees when he was in his 70s. They bothered him to the point that he was having difficulty getting up from a chair. I told him to avoid stress to his knees such as bending them and putting weight on them (for instance, going up and down stairs). I advised that if it was unavoidable to use the stairs he should use the handrails, and when he got up out of a chair he needed to use the armrest. Other examples of stress to the knees include high impact activities such as jumping and running.

I also taught Vernon to do straight-leg-raising exercises, which are very good ways to strengthen the quadriceps muscles. These are the most important muscles for the knees. To do straight-leg-raising exercises, lie on your back keeping one knee bent. You then raise the straight leg two to three inches off the floor and hold it for three to five seconds. Do fifteen to twenty repetitions for a set, at least one set a day. After a while, as the quads get stronger, you may consider doing the straight leg raising with some light ankle weights.

Finally, I told Vernon to gradually work up to walking two miles a day. He was very faithful to the above regimen and within several months, his knee problems dramatically subsided. Vernon actually was in better shape in his 80s than he was in his 70s. So, instead of deteriorating with age he has improved. To this day, at age 91, he has not required any operations on his knees.

Another common orthopedic problem is chronic low back pain. It afflicts many people (unfortunately I am one of them). I have had chronic low back pain for over thirty years. About twenty-five years ago, my back was so bad that at least once a month it would hurt so much that I couldn't stand up straight. This required physical therapy. I began to worry that by the time I reached 40 I would probably be wheelchair bound.

About twenty years ago I started to do three back exercises first thing every morning. These exercises are the pelvic tilt...the knee to the chest stretch...and the partial sit-up. All three of the exercises are done lying flat on the back with the knees bent. Here are some easy instructions to follow:

1. Perform the pelvic tilt by tightening the muscles of your abdomen and flattening your back against the floor. Hold this for two seconds and repeat ten times.

2. Do the knee to chest stretch by pulling each knee to the chest separately with your hand followed by pulling both knees to the chest together. Hold each posture for two seconds and repeat ten times.

3. Finally, do the partial sit-up by sitting up partially and touching each bent knee with the opposite

hand, followed by touching both knees with both hands. Again hold each posture for two seconds and repeat ten times.

These three exercises take less than five minutes to do and help to strengthen and stretch your back before you start the day. I have been religiously doing these exercises daily, having missed only about three to four times over the past twenty years.

My back is now much better. Not only am I not bedridden at the age of 56, I am able to play golf. Additionally, I rarely require physical therapy for my back now. Even though I still have daily pain, I have successfully avoided back surgery so far.

I have been teaching these simple back exercises to my patients for many years. I also teach them to avoid stress to the back, such as bending over to pick up heavy objects. Additionally, I advise them to assume a good posture since this lowers the stress to the back. Many of my patients who follow the above regimen find it very effective.

Let me give you an example. A high-powered CEO came to me with low back pain radiating down her leg. This indicated that there was nerve impingement. She called me to explain her painful symptoms and to request that I refer her to a well-known back specialist she had heard about. I recommended that she come to let me check her out first. After examining her, I recommended a treatment regimen including the daily three back exercises.

She followed my treatment and became pain free. She still does her back exercises daily and is doing well. In fact, she was so impressed with her results that she has been advocating the back exercises to many of her friends.

Before we leave this discussion of the back, I would like to give you another set of very helpful exercises. I call these isometric transverse abdominis exercises. We have all seen weight lifters wearing the wide leather belts to protect their backs. We all have a natural back brace called the transverse abdominis muscles. Strengthen these muscles and you will have a stronger back. Also, if you tighten these muscles while you do lifting or other activities that put stress on the back, it is like wearing a back brace. The following are the steps to learn how to strengthen your transverse abdominis muscles:

1. Pull in your navel with your lower abdominal muscles. These are the transverse abdominis muscles. You can check to see if you are doing this correctly by placing your hands lightly on the lower abdominal wall and feeling the muscles tightening. This can be performed while you are either sitting or standing.

2. Now learn to breathe in and out normally while you are tightening the transverse abdominis muscles. This is important because it allows you to do isometric strengthening of these muscles for

a prolonged period of time without turning blue in the face.

3. Tighten these transverse abdominis muscles and hold for five to ten seconds at a time throughout the day. You can do this sitting down, standing up, driving a car, watching TV, or talking to a friend.

4. Before you do any activity that puts a strain on the back, such as lifting, you should tighten your transverse abdominis muscles. This has a similar effect as wearing a back brace to decrease the chance of hurting your back.

5. The transverse abdominis muscles can also be very helpful in protecting the back in different sports, such as tennis and golf. However, it is important to be able to tighten these muscles without having to think about it and be distracted. This can be accomplished after you have done these exercises so many times that it becomes second nature.

This simple exercise regimen, along with good posture, has helped many of my patients who have back pain. An additional side benefit of these exercises is that you can lose some inches off your waist.

Of course, sometimes orthopedic problems such as severe arthritis or a herniated disc in the back result in excruciating pain down the legs or weakness in the legs. This requires surgical intervention. However, if you follow the above set of principles you can avoid surgery most of the time.

As I said in the beginning of this chapter, it is essential to take care of your joints so that you can avoid injuries and continue to exercise as long as possible.

Chapter **9**
The Stress of Running Behind

Many of my patients tell me that they have a great deal of difficulty trying to lose weight during periods of increased stress. In fact, many people gain a lot of weight when under stress. It is extremely important to reduce stress in order to succeed in losing weight. In this chapter, I will describe an approach to handle a very common type of stress that affects us frequently, the stress of running behind. I am sure most of you have experienced this.

I was under that type of pressure when I served as the Chief of the Medical Staff at Mercy San Juan Hospital in Carmichael, California. This was an extremely demanding position both in terms of time and emotional commitment. I was in charge of several hundred physicians who were staff members of the hospital. I had to attend ten to fifteen meetings a week. I presided over the medical executive committee. I had to handle all of the problems that involved the physicians. This took more than twenty hours a week.

On top of this, I had a full-time solo internal medical practice, which easily averaged sixty hours of work a week. I felt like I had too many things to do but never enough time to do them. Fortunately, I did well surviving the two years as Chief of Staff, and my marriage did not fall apart thanks to Sandy, my loving and tolerant wife of over thirty years. Let me share with you my secret of surviving.

When I set out on a long automobile trip, such as the four-hundred-mile drive from Sacramento to Los Angeles, I dread the long drive. At the beginning of each trip it seems impossible to get there. However, after about the halfway point, I begin to feel a sense of accomplishment and the confidence that I can make it. In other words, when I start thinking of the miles that I have driven already rather than the miles I have yet to drive, I no longer feel overwhelmed.

I applied the above technique to my Chief of Staff years this way. I would divide the day into different tasks. I assigned these tasks to myself arbitrarily. They were not equally difficult, nor did they require equal amounts of time. One example of these tasks was making rounds on my hospitalized patients. This would take between a half hour to several hours. I counted this as one task. Another example was meetings, which typically would take one and a half to two hours. Other tasks were seeing patients in the office in the morning (three to four hours); doing paperwork and phone calls in the morning (one to two hours); seeing patients in the afternoon (three to four hours); doing paperwork and phone calls in the afternoon (one to two hours); and reading EKG's (five to fifteen minutes). Notice that this last task, reading EKG's, takes the least time to accomplish.

I began each day by estimating the number of tasks I had to perform that day. A long and difficult day would be a ten-task day, which usually translated to fifteen to sixteen hours of work. I would then start methodically to perform these tasks, counting only the number of tasks I accomplished, not the number of tasks I had yet to do. I played a mind game with myself by always starting my day by reading EKG's, because after just a few minutes I would have the satisfaction of checking off one task. Using this technique, by early afternoon I would have accomplished perhaps four to five out of eight to ten tasks and would feel like I was half way through, even though I still had eight to nine hours of work left. Like driving to Los Angeles, I would feel that I could make it since I had finished more than 50% of the job. Next thing I knew, I had finished all the tasks.

Using this approach, not only was I able to get everything done, but I also felt the satisfaction of accomplishing something throughout the day. You may say that playing mind games works only for some people and not others. Perhaps that is true, but I think it can work for many people. Let me illustrate by the following example. One day, my office manager came to me bitterly complaining about how much work she had to do and how she did not think she could ever finish it. Her in-laws were visiting, and she had to clean house, cook and get ready for them. She was on the brink of a nervous breakdown.

I told her to take a deep breath, then to divide what she had to do into tasks and concentrate on what she had accomplished rather than what she had yet to do. The next morning, thank God, she showed up to work. I asked her how it went. She replied that she did exactly as I suggested. She actually finished everything and had time to spare.

This approach is very much like the concept of looking at a glass of water as always being half full instead of half empty. The feeling of not having enough time is one of the more common pressures we face and it puts a great deal of stress on all of us. I think you may find this technique helpful in handling the stress of being overwhelmed by too many things to do, and not enough time to do them.

● Steps for Managing Time/Stress

1. List all the tasks you have to do that day.
2. Start with easy-to-accomplish tasks to give yourself momentum.
3. Check off the tasks as you accomplish them.
4. When you finish a little more than 50% of the tasks,

tell yourself you are over half through and that you can finish the rest.

5. Complete the rest of the jobs.

This approach fits perfectly with my daily weight monitoring program. The idea is to not become overwhelmed by the many things you think you have yet to do. If you weigh yourself daily and act to reverse any weight gain, you will only have to deal at the most with 1 to 2 pounds at a time. You can easily manage this. On the other hand, if you do not weigh yourself regularly, you could easily find yourself gaining 5, 10, or even more pounds. Weight gains like this can be overwhelming. This simple method can easily revolutionize the way you approach work and life.

Chapter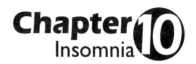
Insomnia

In the last chapter, I discussed the importance of stress reduction in weight loss. Another complaint related to stress is insomnia, a very common problem in this country. It is estimated that insomnia is experienced by nearly one-third of the adult population and is a persistent complaint of about 10%. In this chapter, I will describe my approach to treating it. Insomnia is characterized by complaints of difficulty falling asleep or maintaining sleep, resulting in persistent sleepiness after a night of sleep and impairment of daytime functioning.

First, it is important to identify any underlying causes of insomnia and treat them. These causes include chronic pain, stress, anxiety, depression, certain medications, bladder or prostate problems, neurological problems such as restless leg syndrome, and others.

It is also important to stress that everyone has a different sleep requirement. Some people may get by with four hours of sleep a night while others may need ten. Additionally, some people require less sleep as they get older. Often these people mistake the need for less sleep as insomnia.

For instance, someone who once required eight hours of sleep but now needs only six, would go to bed at 9 p.m. and wake up at 3 a.m., wide awake and unable to go back to sleep. In most cases, he or she would call this insomnia when actually this person had a full night's sleep.

My approach to insomnia (without any correctable underlying causes) is this: I first determine how many hours of sleep that person needs. That is, I estimate the number of hours of continuous sleep needed for that person to feel refreshed in the morning. Let us say this individual estimates he needs seven hours of sleep. I ask what time he wishes to get up in the morning. He says 6 a.m. I then ask that he do the following: get up by 6 a.m. every morning no matter what day of the week it is and no matter how little sleep he has gotten the night before. I ask him to set an alarm clock to accomplish this.

At 6 a.m. he is to open up all the drapes to let the sunlight in or to turn on all the bright lights if it is still dark outside. This will help the sleep center in the brain wake up. He must not take a nap during the day. If he gets drowsy, I tell him to splash cold water on his face. He should avoid caffeine, one of the most common chemicals that causes insomnia. Caffeine can affect people's ability to sleep for up to twelve hours. As few as two to three cups of coffee can significantly disturb sleep in some people. Some other chemicals that can interfere with sleep are alcohol, nicotine, decongestants, cocaine and amphetamines.

I also instruct him to exercise aerobically for at least twenty minutes a day (see Chapter 4 on Exercise for further details). He is to avoid going to bed any earlier than 11 p.m. (11 p.m. to 6 a.m. is seven hours, the amount of sleep he said he needs). If he gets sleepy before 11 p.m. he needs more cold water on his face. By 11 p.m. he may go to bed but only if he is sleepy. He should not go to bed and toss and turn. If this happens, he should get out of bed and read or do something else that doesn't require mental or physical activity.

I ask him to do the same thing if he wakes up in the middle of the night and can't go back to sleep. I also tell him to keep the bedroom nice and quiet and dark because noise and light can interfere with sleep. He should avoid leaving the television on throughout the night. The next morning he is to get up when the alarm clock rings and start the whole routine over again.

The above method may take a few days or weeks to get used to, but it works for most of my patients with insomnia. You need to do all of this to succeed. You cannot sleep in on weekends, take a nap during the day, or drink a lot of caffeine. The method described here is natural, safe and effective.

Now let me give you an example of how this works. A patient, who is a teacher, came to me with a very strange complaint—he had tremendous difficulty with insomnia every year during summer vacation. As soon as school started his problem disappeared. This puzzled him because he really enjoyed summer vacations, when he was free from the pressures of the school year. However, he felt much less relaxed and more stressed when summer ended and school began again, yet he slept much better. This made absolutely no sense to him. He felt it should be the other way around: insomnia during the school year should disappear when summer vacation started.

After closer questioning, I found that he always set the alarm to get up at the same time every morning during the school year. On the other hand, he never set the alarm in the morning during summer vacations. Mystery solved! I recommended that he set his alarm to get up at the same time during his summer vacations. He has not had any problem with insomnia since.

If you are having trouble sleeping, try this method and see if it will work for you. Be sure, however, to follow the instructions in every detail. This is extremely important.

● **To summarize my approach to insomnia:**
1. Check with your doctor to be sure you don't have any treatable underlying condition.

2. Estimate the number of hours of continuous sleep you need to feel rested.
3. Establish the time you wish to get up each morning and set the alarm clock so that you always get up by that time every day.
4. Once you know the time you want to get up, count backwards the number of hours of sleep you need. This will give you the time you should go to bed. Do not go to bed before this time.
5. Avoid forcing sleep (i.e., staying in bed when you can't sleep).
6. Avoid taking a nap during the day.
7. Avoid coffee or other caffeine-containing food or beverages.
8. Avoid alcohol near bedtime: no "night cap."
9. Exercise twenty minutes a day.
10. Keep your bedroom quiet and dark.

Chapter 11
Don't Make Enemies Unnecessarily

As already mentioned, it is difficult to lose weight when you are under a lot of stress. One very common area of stress is the workplace. It is stressful for many people even under the best of circumstances. It is especially taxing if the work environment is hostile. In this chapter I will share with you how to turn potential enemies into friends. Sometimes it is impossible to avoid antagonizing people. However, it is always best to negotiate around problems and avoid making enemies unnecessarily. This was one of my important guiding principles when I was the Chief of the Medical Staff at Mercy San Juan Hospital in the late 1980's.

One illustration of this approach occurred at 4 a.m. one morning. I was awakened by a phone call from a disgruntled neurosurgeon. He was livid about a case he had to take care of in the emergency room. Since there was no urgency, the normal procedure would have been for him to discuss his concerns with me the next day. However, because he was angry, he decided to call me at that ungodly hour while driving home from the hospital just to wake me up. Although I had absolutely nothing to do with the problem that upset him, I kept my cool. I spent about thirty minutes on the phone letting him vent his frustrations and then addressed his concerns by offering possible solutions for the future.

He seemed appeased at the end of the phone call. What was most rewarding was that two days later he called me to apologize for waking me up that morning. We remain friends to this day.

Another example involved the case of an older general practitioner in his 90s, whom I will call Dr. Welby. Dr. Welby had an office practice and also took care of his patients in the hospital and performed surgery. He was still quite sharp mentally—especially for his age—and was capable of taking care of his patients and maintaining their health on an outpatient basis. However, when his patients became sick enough to require hospitalization or surgery, they needed a much higher level of specialized care.

The hospital medical staff was concerned that Dr. Welby's clinical acumen was no longer at the level it needed to be. There was concern that he might compromise the care of patients with acute medical problems that required quick and accurate decision-making. The medical staff planned to monitor Dr. Welby closely and restrict his practice if appropriate. They anticipated that he would probably respond with the normal reaction of anger and defensiveness and even possibly a lawsuit. Of course, as the Chief of the Medical Staff, I was in charge of handling this.

However, as I thought about it, I came up with a different idea. I went to Dr. Welby's office and discussed in a very respectful way the idea of him retiring from the hospital part of his practice. He was quite receptive and agreed to give up hospital work. I then organized a big medical staff party honoring him for all of his past accomplishments, which were many. He was touched at the recognition paid to him by his fellow physicians and gave a moving speech thanking the medical staff for the years they had worked together. He felt proud and honored. Thus what could have been stressful and humiliating for him instead became a positive experience for everyone.

One other example involved my dealings with the head of the legal department of the central organization that managed our hospital. I will call him J.D. Holmes. Mr. Holmes worked at the headquarters in San Francisco and came to Sacramento to meet with us when necessary.

J.D. and I would meet only when there was an impasse between the medical staff and the administration, usually over issues of self-governance of the medical staff. He was like the big gun from out of town brought in by the administration. Needless to say, J.D. and I would meet under adverse situations, always doing battle with each other.

It seemed inevitable that J.D. and I would become bitter enemies. However, to the contrary, we actually became friends. The reason is that we had a lot of mutual respect for each other. We operated under the principle that reasonable people can disagree, and we were always able to find some kind of agreement through compromise at the end of each session.

Our relationship reminded me of the 1957 World War II movie called *The Enemy Below*. It was about an American destroyer captained by Robert Mitchum, and a German submarine under the command of Curt Jurgens. They were engaged in a cat and mouse game trying to destroy each other. At the end of the movie the submarine was so disabled that it had to surface close to the destroyer. As his final act, Kurt Jurgens tried to ram his submarine into the destroyer. This was also the first time the two captains came face-to-face with one another. The captains actually saluted each other, showing their tremendous mutual respect.

I told J.D. about the movie and, to my surprise, he actually rented and enjoyed it. He agreed that the movie reminded him of our relationship. Then we ended up fighting about who was the American Captain and who was the Nazi Captain.

The above illustrates how one can enter into negotiations or even do battle with people without being enemies. This very important principle not only guided me through my term as the Chief of Staff but also has helped me through life.

I mentioned compromise above as an effective tool to negotiation. This is also applicable to dieting and weight control. I am against the uncompromising approach to dieting some people adopt. That is, they absolutely have to avoid certain foods such as ice cream, cookies, candy and fast foods. Many of these people feel deprived all the time. (Also, it can be a pain having them over for dinner because you never know what to serve them.)

I recommend the approach of compromise. You can have almost any kind of food as long as it is not too often and as long as you limit the amount you eat. On the Chang Method of daily weight monitoring, you can occasionally cheat as long as you work on dropping the weight that you gained as a result of cheating, even if it takes a few days. For instance, let's say you are having a birthday party for your child at an ice cream parlor. You suddenly feel an overwhelming urge to have a banana split. What can you do? I suggest you assess carefully how strong this urge is and whether you can suppress it. If you can't, proceed to plan B which is to make a compromise with yourself. Tell yourself to "Go ahead—make my day" and have the banana split. After that, cut down on what you eat the next few days and exercise an additional five to ten minutes each day until the extra weight comes off.

Chapter 12
Don't Jump To Conclusions
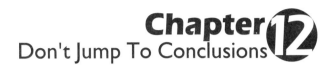

Sometimes things happen which initially appear to have a certain effect but end up by having the opposite effect. In other words, mistakes may end up being opportunities and vice versa. This is certainly true of weight loss.

The Chinese have a well-known story about this. Mr. Choi was a wealthy man in a village many years ago. He owned a beautiful mare that was the envy of everyone. The villagers kept telling Mr. Choi how lucky he was to have such a horse. Mr. Choi replied that maybe this was not such a good thing.

One day someone forgot to close the barn door and the horse escaped. The word spread and the villagers came to offer their sympathy. Mr. Choi responded that maybe that was not such a bad thing.

A few days later the mare returned to Mr. Choi's barn, bringing a stunning stallion with her. Now the villagers came to congratulate Mr. Choi for being so lucky. He merely told them that maybe this was not such a good thing.

Mr. Choi's son trained this amazing stallion. Unfortunately, the stallion threw the son off, breaking his leg. The villagers quickly came to express their condolences. Again, Mr. Choi replied that maybe this was not such a bad thing.

Then a war broke out and all the able bodied young men were drafted. Many lost their lives, but Mr. Choi's son did not have to go due to his injury. By now, I guess you get the point of the story.

Let me give you an example of my own experience that parallels Mr. Choi's story. In June of 1974 my wife and I, along with our five-month-old daughter Lisa, had to drive from California to Fort Riley, Kansas to start my two-year military service. I had just finished my medical residency and we were extremely poor. We had to take the hot and humid southern route (Route 66) because our car did not have enough power to make it over the Rockies. We slept at night in our Volkswagen bus.

Late one night, we arrived at a KOA campground in Amarillo, Texas. It was nearly 9 p.m. and we were starving. We inquired about any nearby place that might be open for food. The camp attendant was very friendly and recommended The Barn, a restaurant about a mile down the road. In fact, she had the menu and showed it to us. The menu listed dishes like escargot and filet mignon at prices way above our budget. We were actually thinking of something more like a fast-food place.

However, it was late and we were desperate so we decided to go ahead and splurge. We then asked the attendant if it was okay for us to go in our tennis shorts. She assured us that it was fine. We did not want to take a chance and changed from shorts into jeans before we went.

As we drove into the parking lot of The Barn in our "hippie car," the Volkswagen bus, we saw many large and expensive cars with long horns on the front fenders and pick-up trucks with gun racks. We felt pretty uncomfortable. This was our very first trip to Texas. We had heard stories of racism. My wife is Caucasian, I am Chinese, and we were not sure how people felt about mixed marriages. We planned our strategy before we went into the restaurant. Actually I did. I told Sandy that we should avoid eye contact and try not to provoke anyone. If someone became hostile, I told Sandy to use Lisa as a shield while I ran for help. (Of course, I was just kidding.)

As we walked into the crowded restaurant, we saw many well-dressed people waiting in the bar to be seated. The men all wore nice western shirts with string ties, big belt buckles and cowboy boots. The women were in colorful dressy outfits. It felt very alien to us. We timidly went up to the hostess and asked if we were dressed appropriately. She told us with a smile that we were fine. We then gave her our names and found a dark quiet corner to wait.

We observed that the people were quite friendly with each other and the atmosphere was festive. There was one middle-aged couple who were especially gregarious. They seemed to know everyone there. The wife had what appeared to be the after effects of Graves Disease. This disease consists of hyperthyroidism due to an overactive goiter (enlarged thyroid gland) and an eye condition called exophthalmos. This means the eyes are bulging and show the whites of the eyes both above and below the iris, resulting in a characteristic stare.

After a while Sandy got up to go to the rest room, leaving me with the baby. I felt uneasy and tried to be as inconspicuous as I could. Next, I noticed that the gregarious lady was staring at us. Then she got up and started towards us. I was panic-stricken and was beginning to feel sorry that we had come, as the villagers in Mr. Choi's story would feel. It turned out that instead of being hostile she was actually admiring our beautiful baby!

She introduced herself as Sue and her husband as Bill. Sandy returned and we started a friendly conversation. Then Sue suggested that we join them since they were practically next in line for a table. We thanked them and the next thing we knew, we were given the best table in the house—one with lots of privacy as well as a place to put little Lisa down for a nap. At this point we felt very lucky that we had come, as the villagers would feel in Mr. Choi's story.

Before we ordered the food, Sue asked if we had ever had a "Mai Tai" before. We responded that we had, in California. Sue told us the Mai Tais there were really good and probably larger than any we had in California. She insisted that we try one. You have to understand, we were on a limited budget and were not big drinkers. However, out of politeness, we ordered a Texas-sized Mai Tai for Sandy. It turned out to be the largest Mai Tai I had ever seen. The glass was so tall that, with the straw, Sandy had to stand up to drink it. It was not watered down and, halfway through the Mai Tai, Sandy's chin was resting on the table.

Next came the menu. Bill asked if we had ever tried "mountain oysters." We said we hadn't. He explained that they were sheep testicles, a real Texas delicacy. He told us this restaurant had the absolute best mountain oysters anywhere. He insisted that we try them. I swallowed hard and ordered the mountain oysters. The same went for the entrees. We were forced to order the filet mignon. Basically, we were pressured into ordering food far more expensive than we could afford. The food (except for the mountain oysters) was good and the company was delightful. However, we felt anxious because we were going to have to really tighten our belts for the rest of the trip. Unlucky, as Mr. Choi's villagers would say.

After dinner the waitress came and asked if she

should prepare two checks or one. Sandy and I, of course, said "two." Bill asked for one check. Sue and Bill insisted on treating us because we were guests to their city and to Texas. They merely urged us to pass the favor along to someone else in the future. We were dumbfounded by the generosity of these strangers and felt lucky again.

Like Mr. Choi's story, our evening was filled with ups and downs in our emotions, but ended happily. The take-home lesson is to not jump to conclusions. Take time to evaluate the situation and try to make the best of it, as Mr. Choi did.

This principle is applicable to my daily weight monitoring program. One major reason that many people do not weigh themselves regularly is that they are afraid they might find that they have gained weight.

Is it good or is it bad to discover this? Although most people think it is bad, I look upon it as something good. This is because you can easily reverse a small weight gain if you know about it and act immediately. Simply eat less for a few days and you have undone the damage. This is far better than not discovering the weight gain until it is so large that it becomes a major project to correct.

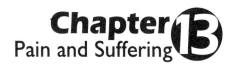

Chapter 13
Pain and Suffering

The part of my weight loss program that is most difficult to carry out is the **Weight Reduction Mode**. There is going to be some short-term pain and suffering involved during this phase. I suggest limiting the duration of this mode to a set time period such as one month. It is easier to endure suffering for a pre-determined, temporary period rather than forever. Let me describe some principles that I find helpful in reducing the pain and suffering we face in our daily lives. These principles can also be used to help us to lose weight.

PRINCIPLE 1: Know that the suffering is temporary.

The amount of pain a person can endure depends on several factors: (1) an individual's pain threshold, (2) the intensity of the pain and (3) the duration of the pain. The duration of the pain is extremely important. For example, when I do a biopsy of a patient's skin lesion I give a local anesthetic in the form of a shot to numb it. The shot is intensely painful. However, I warn my patients beforehand that it will hurt, but only for a moment. So far, no one has ever had a problem handling this short-lived, but intense, pain.

Let me further illustrate this principle with some of my own experiences. One of the most difficult periods of my life occurred during my internship, just after I finished medical school. I was on call for twenty-four hours every third day and sometimes every second day, depending on the rotation. Here is how the every-third-day call worked. On the first day I was in the hospital all day taking care of sick patients. That night I stayed in the hospital to admit patients who needed to be hospitalized. Most of these patients were extremely ill, requiring a tremendous amount of care and worry. I would get very little sleep that night, perhaps two to three hours at the most. On the second day I would work the whole day, often finishing at midnight. I would then go home and sleep. The third day was the best because, even though I had to work twelve to fourteen hours, at least I had gotten a few hours of sleep the night before and I was able to go home to sleep that night.

However, on that third day all I could think about was the next day when the cycle would start all over again with the murderous twenty-four-hour call. Remember, this was an every-third-day call schedule. It was much worse when I had the every-second-day call schedule. How did I survive my internship? With great difficulty. Needless to say, I did not do much of anything other than go to work, come home, sleep, and go back to work again.

I remember one of the rare occasions when my wife and I went out to dinner because a very close childhood friend of hers was visiting from out of town. The bill came after dinner and I started to check the total. My wife began to worry when I kept staring at the check without moving. She was worried that I was upset about the bill. Remember, we were living on an intern's salary that was less than the minimum wage. However, when she talked to me I came to with a start. It turned out that I was so exhausted I had fallen asleep while adding up the bill!

Another incident that sticks in my mind happened one night when I was treating an elderly gentleman with severe breathing problems due to his lung disease. He was on the verge of needing to be put on a respirator, and I had to watch him very closely. I had been up for about twenty hours and was exhausted. I am not one to cry easily. In fact, at that point in my life I had not cried for almost twenty years, since I was six years old. However that night, while I was at this very sick patient's bedside, I was so exhausted physically and so mentally drained that I felt like crying. Fortunately, I was able to fight back the tears. Imagine how scary it would have been for that poor gentleman, struggling for his life, to see his doctor breaking down in front of him!

As you can see, my internship was a very difficult year. One thing that helped me get through it was the fact that I knew it was not permanent. So the principle here is that generally we can handle pain and suffering better if we know that they won't last forever, that they will end some day. This principle is the reason why I recommend that the **Weight Reduction Mode** be limited to thirty days at a time.

PRINCIPLE 2: Times were much harder in the past, or "This is nothing compared to..."

How happy or how miserable we feel often depends on whom we compare ourselves to. For example, a person who makes $30 an hour will feel happy and content if he compares himself to a person at a fast food place earning minimum wage. On the other hand, he will be miserable and dissatisfied if he compares himself to a trial lawyer who makes $400 an hour.

When it comes to pain and suffering, the same principle applies. If we remember back to periods in our lives when we experienced severe suffering, it can make the present suffering seem more tolerable. Here is an example from my past experiences.

After my internship, I completed two years of residency in Internal Medicine. It was pretty grueling but better than internship. I again used the method of handling the stress by telling myself that, "This will not last forever!" Another powerful weapon I used to survive residency was to remember how much harder internship had been. To borrow a phrase from Dustin Hoffman in the movie *Wag the Dog*, "This is nothing!" With the help of these principles I survived and eventually finished all of my training.

Next, I went into the Army and completed my two years of military service at Fort Riley, Kansas. Those two years in the military were much easier than the previous years of internship and residency training. I did not have to use any of the above rationalizations to help me through.

Then came private practice, which was extremely busy. This was especially true when I served as the Chief of the Medical Staff at the hospital while handling a solo private practice. I routinely worked seventy to eighty hours a week. How did I handle this? I used the same principles as above, constantly telling myself that the Chief of Staff position would be over in two years and reminding myself that internship had been much harder.

How does this apply to weight loss? During the **Weight Reduction Mode,** or the "suffering phase" for those of you who have starved yourselves to lose weight in the past, say to yourselves, "This is nothing! I have lost much more than five pounds before." If you have never gone through the process of trying to lose weight in the past, think of some other painful period in your life that you endured and survived. If you can remember this, you will have a good chance of succeeding.

PRINCIPLE 3: Positive thinking: it is easy, you can do it!

This is undoubtedly the guiding principle for most successful people in the past and the present. One personal experience I'd like to share with you is the example of my father, who went from being the poorest of the poor, a peasant in China in the early 1900's, to being very successful in America. Here is his story.

My father was born in a village in southern China to a poor peasant family. He was the oldest of five children. At the age of thirteen, he was forced to leave home because they were unable to feed him any more. He had to take a long boat trip to Shanghai, where his grandfather worked. He traveled on a livestock boat and slept with the pigs. He was alone and scared, clutching the wooden box that held all of his earthly possessions. The miserable journey lasted many days. He was not sure that he would survive the trip.

My father had no money and did not speak the Shanghainese dialect. Luckily he found his grandfather, who worked at a small hotel. He put my father up in a room where the hotel workers lived. It was a tiny room with poor lighting, crowded with a dozen or so men who smoked opium whenever they had the chance. These men were desperately poor with no future and escaped their hopeless lives by smoking opium. They encouraged my father to do the same.

However, my father was a man of courage and

vision even at that young age. He accomplished many things and surmounted unbelievable hardships. He became very successful because he was willing to work incredibly hard and had no fear of failure. He was fully confident that he could achieve whatever he wanted to.

Instead of smoking opium, my father found a job as an apprentice in a printing shop making $5 a month. He would walk several miles to work just to save a penny so that he could send money to his family back in the village.

My father never had any formal education, yet he learned multiple Chinese dialects including Cantonese, Mandarin, and Shanghainese, as well as English. He knew that these languages were crucial if he wanted to be successful. His next job was at a newspaper company. He kept advancing in his career. In his early 20s he got a job at the government Foreign Affairs Office because of his proficiency in multiple languages, especially English. He then moved to Chunking, China's new capitol. There my father met a beautiful young maiden, triumphed over all the other suitors, and married my mother. (My mother turned 81 recently and looks like she could be my older sister. What is her secret to staying so young? She exercises and weighs herself every day.)

A better opportunity came up at CNAC (China Airlines) and my father applied for the job along with over a thousand other applicants. He got the job and we moved to India. My father worked hard and saved a bit of money. A few years later, after World War II ended, our family moved back to China. My father became a very successful businessman and bought a beautiful three-story house in Tianjin, a city not far from Beijing.

Unfortunately, the Communists took over. Gradually, things got worse and worse. A friend, at the risk of his own life, secretly warned my father that a purge against landowners and business people was coming. My father knew he could not take the whole family out of Communist China. With much difficulty and in the guise of a business trip, he escaped to Hong Kong without his family and with almost no money. There he lived at the YMCA and struggled to make a living.

Thousands of people had escaped to Hong Kong and could not earn enough to live on or to get their families out of China. People were desperate. My father described well-educated people picking up cigarette butts on the street to earn a little money. Many lost all hope and committed suicide. One evening at the YMCA, my father played chess with a friend who seemed to be his usual self. Sadly, later that night, the friend went to the roof of the building, put a paper sack over his head, and jumped to his death. Such stories were commonplace.

My father refused to give up. He survived and, after a few years, made enough money to pay the Communist government to ransom us out of China. This depleted all of his savings and he had to start over again. He worked several different jobs until a golden opportunity at Pan

American Airways in Hong Kong opened up. Again, thousands of people applied for this coveted job. My father got it.

He worked for Pan American Airways for a few years, and we lived a good life. However, he knew that opportunities in Hong Kong would be limited for his children. He saw America as the land of freedom and opportunity and wanted to move here. Such a move was risky because he didn't know anyone in this country. Unfortunately, his job at Pan American was not transferable. However, he knew the move was very important to his children's future.

A wonderful chance came when the American government under President Eisenhower opened up extra immigration slots for refugees from Communist China. After months of applying, we were finally accepted. In 1959, our family of five immigrated to this country from Hong Kong.

When we arrived in the United States, my father did not have a job, and the money he had did not go very far due to the unfavorable seven to one exchange rate. He was unfazed. He went door to door and found a job in a bank as a teller making $200 a month. Our family of five lived in a tiny one-bedroom apartment over a garage.

He eventually got a job with Pan American again and worked there until he retired. While working at Pan Am he studied hard to obtain a real estate license.

This was extremely difficult because of the mathematics involved. He had never studied mathematics before. Also he was working sixteen hours a day at Pan Am. With the perseverance so typical of him, he passed the exam and got his real estate license. He then sold real estate on weekends. As time passed, he became a real estate broker and invested in real estate. By the time my father retired he was quite successful.

My father started out as a poor peasant boy in China with no formal education and few opportunities. Yet he learned multiple languages, became very successful despite multiple major set backs, and brought up three sons who all went to college. What was his secret formula? There were many factors including hard work, perseverance, focus, and tremendous foresight. However, I believe the most important trait my father had was positive thinking. He knew that he could accomplish whatever he wanted to do. He always said that the word "difficult" did not exist.

When it comes to weight loss, the same principle applies. Think positively and know that you can do it.

PRINCIPLE 4: Know that the goal is worthwhile.

All Olympic competitors illustrate this principle. These fine athletes go through tremendous amounts of pain and suffering during their training. They are able to accomplish this because they are working toward the noble goal of competing against the best athletes in the world.

Another phenomenon that involves pain and suffering is childbirth. Many women endure pain—some endure a great deal of pain—but most mothers, in my experience, feel that the new baby that they hold in their arms makes the suffering worthwhile. In a way, the weight loss process is like childbirth. You go through a certain amount of pain and suffering to bring out a new you, a happier and healthier you. Is it a worthwhile cause? I certainly think so.

Chapter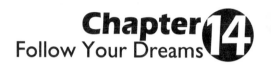
Follow Your Dreams

I wanted to be a doctor ever since I was in grade school. I had to work hard to achieve this goal and I feel fortunate that I was able to reach it. Since childhood I've also had the secret dream of becoming a rock star. I remember in Hong Kong, at the age of nine or ten, I would strum a badminton racket and pretend that I was Elvis Presley.

I started my private practice in 1976 at Mercy San Juan Hospital in Carmichael, California. There was an annual charity event for the near-by Mercy High School featuring the physicians at the hospital playing basketball against our good friends the attorneys. I came up with the idea of forming a band consisting of four doctors performing 50's songs at the end of the annual basketball games. We thought of names for the group such as the "Four Skins," but decided that it sounded too clinical. We ended up calling ourselves Doc Rock. I chose only easy "Doo Wop" songs from the 50's, which were fun and relatively easy to perform. Even so, we had to practice long and hard because we were all novices without any previous experience. In our first year's performance, we played only six songs and sounded pretty bad. However, our audience was large and quite enthusiastic. We even had screaming women—mostly nurses at the hospital—rushing the stage. It was one of the most enjoyable and most exciting things that I have done in my life. I felt like a super star.

We continued to perform yearly and gradually sounded better. Our repertoire also expanded. In 1984, we were featured on "Weeknights," a weekly television news magazine featuring three ten-minute stories each week. We were first filmed in our suits examining patients at the hospital. Then the scene switched to us all greased up playing Rock and Roll music. I looked like Bowser in the group Sha Na Na. I had my hair greased up and wore jeans and a T-shirt with a pack of cigarettes rolled up in the sleeve. (I had to borrow the cigarettes.) I even had tattoos on my arms with a skull on one side and "Mom" on the other. Actually, I looked far meaner than Bowser. The "Weeknights" show was so successful that my office was bombarded with phone calls from people requesting Doc Rock to perform for them. Incidentally, we made the "Best of Weeknights" at the end of the year featuring three of the top rated "Weeknights" shows in 1984.

Like many successful bands in history, we were

unable to stay together forever. Our last Doc Rock performance took place in 1985. I went out with a bang. I changed from my traditional Sha Na Na look to a punk rocker's look. I had a Mohawk hairdo, with gold on the top and blue and red on each side. My face was painted white with an arrow diagonally across. I put on black lipstick and wore a black shirt with zippers randomly placed all over. When unzipped, it gave the appearance of a shirt torn in many places. I wore a pair of fake black leather pants and leather-studded wristbands. I had on a pair of high top canvas tennis shoes with about ten horizontal stripes in rainbow colors. I had a lot of fun shopping for the outfit and you can imagine what the salespeople thought. They undoubtedly decided I was going through a severe midlife crisis.

Our last performance was a smash hit. The whole experience was a total fantasy come true, a dream realized. I hope you can take from this the message that it is a wonderful thing to have dreams in life and to never stop pursuing them.

An interesting follow up story on my rock and roll career occurred in 1994. The Sacramento El Dorado Medical Society holds its annual new officers' induction dinner every January. In 1994, the new president of the society decided to have a doctors' talent show at the induction dinner that year.

I received a call from the social committee chairwoman one day, asking about our Doc Rock group that she had heard so much about. She was hoping that we could perform at the talent show. I thanked her for her interest and told her that, sadly, Doc Rock had disbanded several years before. After talking to her for a while, we decided that I could enter the talent show alone, doing something like karaoke. I decided to sing one of my all time favorite "Doo Wop" songs, "In the Still of The Night," by the Five Satins. I recruited a group and we called ourselves *Henry Chang and the Sidekicks*. For the next few weeks, with the help of my wife who came up with the idea of the show and helped to choreograph it, we rehearsed intensely.

The big event took place in January 1994 at the Grand Ballroom of the Hyatt Regency Hotel in Sacramento. It was a black-tie affair with over two hundred doctors and their guests. Most of the doctors in the talent show did very cultured performances such as classical music on the violin, jazz piano pieces and a barbershop quartet. Then came my number. I strolled onto the stage wearing a Hawaiian shirt, white shorts and no shoes. Accompanying me was a beautiful 19-year-old young lady with long blond hair wearing a short white sun dress. Her name was Kim. Three tough-looking guys who were the back-up singers followed us.

I helped Kim to sit on a stool beside me and gave her a rose. I then proceeded to sing "In The Still of The Night" while Kim and I looked at each other romantically. In the middle of the song, during the saxophone interlude,

I signaled to my back-up singers to come forward holding a one-inch thick pine wood board. I first did a sidekick and broke the board. I turned to Kim and asked her if she was impressed. She shook her head coyly to signal "no." The guys then held out another board and I promptly broke it with a palm strike. I looked at Kim again and asked, "Now are you impressed?" She again shook her head. Finally, the guys brought out a third board and held it high above my head. I did a jumping front kick and with surgical-like precision broke the board again. I then did a Jimmy Connor fist pump and resumed singing the second half of the song. At this point the back-up singers went from the Four Tops type of moves to doing sidekicks in the background. The audience roared in laughter. I was very full of myself and was flexing my biceps as I was singing. Kim was now looking more and more annoyed.

As I was finishing the song, Kim got up from the stool and signaled to the guys to bring out a board. I asked her, "What do you think you are doing? You can't break that board. You are a girl!" On that note Kim put the rose in her teeth, grabbed the board from the guys and broke it with her head! She then gave a Jimmy Connor fist pump, took the rose from her teeth, flung it across the room and stormed off the stage while I was finishing my song. My back-up singers eagerly followed Kim, leaving me all by myself holding the microphone.

I then introduced the audience to my three back-up singers. They were all Tai Kwon Do experts. Two of them were first degree black belts and the other was a third degree black belt. Finally, I introduced the lovely young lady as Kim, a second degree black belt and martial arts instructor. I joked that she was also known as the "Mistress of Death."

The entire act lasted about four minutes. As far as I know, it was the only performance ever to combine these two arts: singing and martial arts.

I am sure many of you have dreamed about losing weight so that you could feel better both physically and emotionally. Unfortunately, too many of you have lost weight in the past and then gained it all back within a few months, shattering your dreams entirely. If this has been happening to you over and over, you don't have to put up with it any longer.

The good news is that you can have your dream of permanent weight loss come true by following my simple and effective daily monitoring program. You can take weight off and keep it off. Dreams do come true.

Chapter 15
Happiness

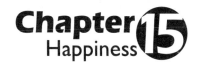

People are unlikely to succeed at anything unless they enjoy doing it. Weight loss is no exception. People who are happy during the process of weight reduction have a much higher chance of success.

Happiness has nothing to do with what you have. It is not related to how much money you have, how big your house is, what kind of car you drive, how important the job you hold or, for you golfers, how low your handicap is. I know of a few wealthy CEO's who live in big houses and have low golf handicaps and are not happy.

Happiness is within you. It is how you feel about yourself. No matter how many assets you have, there are always people who have more. At this moment, Bill Gates is about the only exception. If you compare yourself to more wealthy people, you'll always feel poor and unhappy. By the same token, there are always people who have less.

I visited the Mayan ruins in Mexico recently and saw one of the huts the Mayan people lived in. It was about the size of a large bathroom. The walls were made of straw and mud, and it had a thatch roof. The bed was a hammock stretched across the hut at night. There was no electricity or running water. The tour guide told us that the people still live this way today and are happy. Imagine our American teenagers living under these conditions, especially without their televisions or video games. Happiness is not defined by the absolute amount of money or materialistic possessions you have. It is how you feel about yourself.

Several years ago I played a lot of tennis and was getting to be reasonably good for a beginner. However, my game was up and down. I would play well some days but not so well on others. When I was not playing well, it affected my entire outlook on life. I felt dejected and unhappy. During one of those periods when I was playing tennis poorly and feeling sorry for myself, I found myself making rounds on a patient of mine in the hospital. She was in her 70s and had a broken hip that was fixed with a pin.

Unfortunately, she had another bad fall and broke the pin. The damage was so severe that it was not possible to fix it. She would never walk again. When I saw her that day in the hospital, she had been bedridden for many days due to this tragic injury. I felt sorry for her. When I asked how she felt, she replied cheerfully that she just woke up from one of the most wonderful dreams. She dreamt that she took a step, and she was so happy. When I heard that, I was overwhelmed with shame. Here I was, young and healthy and able to run and jump and play a vigorous game of tennis, yet I was unhappy and felt sorry for myself because my game was not quite up to par. On the other hand, here was a woman who could only dream about taking one step and she was happy about this. From that moment on I stopped feeling unhappy about how I played tennis.

Here's one more unbelievable example about how one finds happiness. One day I walked into the examination room to see a patient whom I will call Theresa. She contracted polio at the age of three. Her childhood polio unfortunately had left her a quadriplegic. She could no longer use her arms and legs. She was completely paralyzed from her neck down. About the only thing she could do was to move her head up-and-down and side-to-side. In fact, if you moved her body forward while she was sitting up she was unable to move it back herself.

Theresa was in her 30s when I first met her. She was in her wheelchair. Her head was the size of a normal 30-year-old person. Her body was the size of a 5 year old. Her arms and legs had withered away from disuse.

I was stunned by Theresa's appearance. I was even more surprised to see her in the examination room all by herself, without anyone to help her or to interpret for her.

Theresa greeted me with an enthusiastic smile. It turned out that she was a delightful, extremely intelligent, and independent woman. She used an electrically motorized wheel chair that had switches that she controlled skillfully with her teeth. She was pleasant and articulate.

Theresa worked full-time as an advocate for the disabled. My first question was how did she write? I soon found out that she wrote with her teeth. Her "tooth writing" was beautiful and much better than my handwriting. I also found out that instead of staying home and feeling sorry for herself, Theresa went to school just like everybody else. After high school, she went on to college and got her bachelor's and master's degrees. On top of everything, she was bilingual, fluent in both Spanish and English.

I was absolutely overwhelmed by the amazing achievement of this courageous woman. She was very easy and pleasant to talk with. I quickly forgot that she looked different from everyone else. This apparently was how our state legislators felt when she came before them to plead for better legislation to help the disabled. The result was that Theresa almost single-handedly helped pass some of the most progressive laws for the disabled in California.

Now, with this tragic illness that caused her to be so severely handicapped, was Theresa happy or sad? The answer was unequivocally that she was happy. She was cheerful and enthusiastic. She never felt sorry for herself. She loved her job. She surrounded herself with people she loved and who loved her. She would not take any time off even when she was sick. At the end she was so sick that she had to be brought from work straight to the emergency room, and she was admitted directly to the intensive care unit because she could not breathe. Unfortunately, her polio was so advanced that it caused her lungs to fail. She never made it out of the hospital. I felt terrible about Theresa's death. Our entire community suffered greatly from the loss of such a remarkable person.

Theresa was undoubtedly the most inspirational person I have ever met. She demonstrated that you can overcome just about any degree of disability by sheer determination. She also showed us that you can be happy and enjoy life despite overwhelming hardship and adversity.

Now, let's go back to weight loss and the concept of happiness. First, let's analyze why most people fail to lose weight and keep it off. One important reason is that most people begin by being unhappy about their weight, unlike Theresa, who felt happy about herself. As a result of this unhappiness, these people are impatient and feel like failures if their weight doesn't drop rapidly, on a daily basis. They go on extremely restrictive diets, deny themselves all kinds of food, and feel deprived and unhappy all the time. They also can't bear to weigh themselves every day for fear they won't lose weight fast enough. Because of this, they are unwilling to monitor their daily progress.

Additionally, most people set unrealistic weight goals. They would like to take off 20% to 30% of their weight all at once. Even if they succeed, they are so miserable doing this that most of them revert right back to their previous lifestyle and eventually gain all the weight back.

On the other hand, the Chang Method differs by starting you out in the **Weight Maintenance Mode,** where it is not important to lose weight immediately. It stresses that you are *successful* if you can maintain this weight. As a result, you should not be afraid to weigh yourself every day. In fact, you should be eager to do so because this is the best way to maintain your weight.

When you get the knack of the **Weight Maintenance Mode,** you are then ready for the **Weight Reduction Mode**. Here you will choose a realistic weight-loss goal such as 5 pounds over a thirty-day period. You know that even this relatively small amount of weight loss will benefit your health significantly. Above all, you know that once you achieve this goal you will be able to maintain the hard-fought weight loss **forever**.

So you see, with the Chang Method you will always feel positive and successful. As a result, you will enjoy the process of losing weight. Again, remember that we are unlikely to succeed in doing anything unless we enjoy doing it.

Chapter 16
How I Approach My Patients About Daily Weighing

I will start by asking two simple questions.

1. Would you like to lose some weight and keep it off?
   (Answer: Of course.)
2. Have you ever gone on a diet, lost a whole bunch of weight, but then gained it all back?
   (Answer: Yes, many times.)

You are not the only one who has done this. Over 95% of the people who succeed in losing weight gain it back. This makes it almost not worthwhile to work so hard to lose the weight when you know that there is less than 5% chance that you will succeed in keeping it off.

In this chapter, I am going to review what I have been telling you throughout this book. I want to emphasize again the importance of weight maintenance and go back over how to do it easily without pain.

As we have seen, it is very hard to lose weight and keep it off because the body acts like a thermostat set at the highest weight you've attained. So, let's say your highest weight is 200 pounds. The body always wants to come back to this weight. Whether you lose 10, 20, or 50 pounds, the body always wants to end up at 200 pounds, however long it takes—a week, a month, or a year. Just like when you set your home thermostat at eighty degrees, the temperature will eventually climb to eighty degrees. The body also responds this way. To add insult to injury, we all have a tendency to gain weight as we get older, and the thermostat keeps re-setting to the higher weight. So you see, trying to lose weight is an uphill battle all the way.

Now, how can you win this war against weight gain? The answer, I emphasize again in this chapter, is weighing yourself every day. You need to get a scale. Be sure the scale is accurate. Accurate doesn't mean it has to correlate exactly with your doctor's office scale. Accurate means that if you get on it three times in a row, it gives the same reading, with no more than half a pound difference.

● To Summarize
- Be sure to have a reliable scale and weigh yourself once a day at the same time.
- Start with the **Weight Maintenance Mode**. Keep from gaining any weight by acting on any weight gain you detect from one day to the next. Be patient

because it may take a few days to drop the pound or two that you gained. Feel like a success if you are able to maintain your weight.

- After a period of successful weight maintenance, start on the **Weight Reduction Mode.** Set a realistic goal such as losing 5 pounds over a month. Think of it as a temporary sacrifice for a healthier future life.
- Once you achieve this goal, get right back on the **Weight Maintenance Mode** so that you will never gain the weight back.
- Repeat this small weight loss as many times as you need to reach your final weight loss goal. You may have set this at 20 pounds. This will require you to repeat your weight loss month three more times.
- Get back on the **Weight Maintenance Mode** when you feel that you have reached your final goal weight. You will remain on this mode forever, weighing yourself everyday.

Now you are ready to join the growing number of people who not only lose weight, but also keep it off forever. As shown by the experiences of my own overweight patients, the Chang Method works. If you will follow the instructions exactly, it will work for you. I have great hopes for you. I know you can do it. May you become healthy, trim, and ready to enjoy life to its fullest.

Appendix A
The Support for Daily Weight Monitoring

Is there proof that daily weight monitoring works in helping people lose weight and keep it off? Yes, there is both my original study involving 140 patients and the National Weight Control Registry study.

My study is ongoing and this book is the first report of it. For the last year I have been counseling my patients about weight reduction using the Chang Method (discussed in Chapter 2). So far, a total of 140 patients (68 females, 72 males) have followed my daily weighing regimen. The average age of the group was 59 years old, the average weight at the onset was 214 pounds, and the average length of participation was six months.

I did not anticipate any dramatic success in promoting weight loss since I took only five to ten minutes at the end of a regular office visit to talk about the daily monitoring program. I did not offer any special diets or spend time talking about exercise. I did not conduct special follow-up visits or even phone calls except for the next regular office visit for the patient's usual medical problems. This is in contrast to all the other diet programs or studies, where the participants have frequent visits with case managers or dietitians. My hope at the beginning of the study was that this simple method would help a majority of patients maintain their weight and not gain. I would have been very pleased if even a few of them lost some weight.

To my amazement the results were overwhelmingly positive...130 of the 140 patients lost weight (see Table 1). This was a whopping 93% of the group. The average weight loss over six months was 10.3 pounds. Three of the 140 patients had no weight change. Only 7 of the 140 patients gained weight (see Table 2). However, some of these seeming "failures" were actually successes. One woman followed my program for two months but gained a pound. I found out that she went from getting no exercise to rowing one and a half hours three times a week with the women's rowing team. Even though I list her as a weight loss "failure" in my study, she was actually a success because she gained muscle weight and lost fat.

I was astonished that such a high percentage of my patients succeeded in losing so many pounds. What is even more rewarding is that they were enthusiastic about weighing themselves daily. They found it easy to do and it gave them confidence that they could lose more weight and maintain the weight loss. None of them was demoralized or frustrated by daily weighing. Many of them thanked me profusely for directing them to this approach and wondered why no one else had told them about this before. They felt that they could stay on this program forever and they felt great!

Jason, who lost 20 pounds in two months, wrote: "When Dr. Chang told me that in order to lose weight, I needed to weigh myself every day, I did not understand why. But after the first couple of months of weighing myself every day, the benefits were obvious. It was easy to see if what I was doing every day was helping me to lose the weight. I will be weighing myself everyday for the rest of my life. Thanks, Dr. Chang."

Ken wrote: "I find Dr. Chang's program very effective and easy to follow. It does not require taking any medication or any special regimen...Thank you for your excellent program."

Isabelle found my program to be tremendously helpful, having lost 23 pounds in nine months, and wrote: "Through the guidance from Dr. Chang, I have embarked on a program to lose weight and improve my health. I have followed his instructions on weighing myself daily. This has been a tremendous help. Those extra pounds can add up very quickly when you are not keeping track. I can make little daily adjustments in my food intake to make sure I stay on track. Thanks to Dr. Chang's advice and encouragement I am losing weight and keeping it off."

Table 1 – Positive Patient Results Using the Chang Method

	Age	Start Weight	End Weight	Change in Lbs.	Percent Change	Start Date	End Date	Time In Months
1	60	226	175	51	22.57%	Jan-03	Jul-03	6
2	78	187	181	6	3.21%	Jul-02	May-03	10
3	62	223	215	8	3.59%	Dec-02	Feb-03	2
4	58	209	200	9	4.31%	Aug-02	Feb-03	6
5	63	229	216	13	5.68%	Feb-02	Aug-02	6
6	54	228.5	221	7.5	3.28%	Apr-03	Jun-03	2
7	61	179	168	11	6.15%	Apr-02	Oct-02	6
8	68	164	157	7	4.27%	Aug-02	Apr-03	8
9	68	254	240	14	5.51%	Jul-02	Dec-02	5
10	25	213	208	5	2.35%	May-02	Jul-02	2
11	59	138	129	9	6.52%	Jul-02	Feb-03	7
12	68	189	188	1	0.53%	Oct-02	May-03	7
13	47	264	255.5	8.5	3.22%	Mar-03	Jun-03	3
14	57	230	229	1	0.43%	Jun-02	May-03	11
15	50	181	174	7	3.87%	Nov-02	Jun-03	7
16	39	236	224	12	5.08%	Mar-02	Jul-02	4
17	70	256	253	3	1.17%	Dec-02	Apr-03	4
18	44	215	209	6	2.79%	Mar-03	Apr-03	1
19	64	201	191.5	9.5	4.73%	Nov-02	Mar-03	4
20	75	219	211	8	3.65%	Apr-02	Oct-02	6
21	71	230	210	20	8.70%	Apr-02	Jul-02	3
22	69	181	177.5	3.5	1.93%	Feb-03	May-03	3
23	46	217	210	7	3.23%	Apr-02	Oct-02	6
24	33	250	247	3	1.20%	Dec-02	Feb-03	2
25	80	201	188	13	6.47%	May-02	Apr-03	11
26	71	236	227	9	3.81%	Oct-02	Apr-03	6
27	31	211	209.5	1.5	0.71%	May-03	Jun-03	1
28	50	148	144	4	2.70%	Jul-02	Oct-02	3
29	62	208	197	11	5.29%	May-02	Dec-02	7
30	63	168	163	5	2.98%	Oct-02	Apr-03	6
31	69	234	209	25	10.68%	May-02	Jun-03	13
32	51	284.5	255.5	29	10.19%	Jun-02	Nov-02	5
33	53	230	212	18	7.83%	Aug-02	Jan-03	5

	Age	Start Weight	End Weight	Change in Lbs.	Percent Change	Start Date	End Date	Time In Months
								Table 1 – Positive Patient Results Using the Chang Method (continued)
34	54	270	244	26	9.63%	Apr-02	Apr-03	12
35	50	192	185	7	3.65%	Nov-02	Feb-03	3
36	72	216.5	206	10.5	4.85%	Sep-02	Feb-03	5
37	54	312	310	2	0.64%	Aug-02	Sep-02	1
38	54	204	203	1	0.49%	May-02	Feb-03	9
39	34	207	198	9	4.35%	May-02	Nov-02	6
40	75	184	172	12	6.52%	Dec-02	Jun-03	6
41	41	214	209	5	2.34%	Feb-03	May-03	3
42	56	206	200	6	2.91%	Jun-02	Dec-02	6
43	49	248	219	29	11.69%	Oct-02	Jun-03	8
44	52	262	255	7	2.67%	Jul-02	Nov-02	4
45	51	178	174	4	2.25%	Jun-02	Jan-03	7
46	65	214	202	12	5.61%	Jul-02	Apr-03	9
47	52	175	170.5	4.5	2.57%	Aug-02	Oct-02	2
48	24	241	220	21	8.71%	Oct-02	Feb-03	4
49	64	190	184.5	5.5	2.89%	Aug-02	Feb-03	6
50	74	246	240	6	2.44%	Aug-02	Dec-02	4
51	54	241.5	236	5.5	2.28%	Apr-02	Jul-02	3
52	71	153	150	3	1.96%	Nov-02	Feb-03	3
53	62	169	163	6	3.55%	Apr-02	Jul-02	3
54	83	181	159	22	12.15%	Feb-03	Jun-03	4
55	57	233	218	15	6.44%	Sep-02	Jun-03	9
56	54	172	170	2	1.16%	Apr-02	Apr-03	12
57	66	190	182	8	4.21%	Nov-02	May-03	6
58	68	244	228	16	6.56%	Jan-03	Mar-03	2
59	68	161	154	7	4.35%	Jun-02	Feb-03	8
60	49	173	139	34	19.65%	Aug-01	Aug-02	12
61	59	270	264	6	2.22%	Nov-02	Feb-03	3
62	61	243	239	4	1.65%	Jul-02	Sep-02	2
63	61	160.5	147	13.5	8.41%	May-02	Oct-02	5
64	19	168	153	15	8.93%	Apr-02	Apr-03	12
65	57	191	188	3	1.57%	Jun-02	Jul-02	1
66	40	242	236	6	2.48%	Aug-02	Mar-03	7

	Age	Start Weight	End Weight	Change in Lbs.	Percent Change	Start Date	End Date	Time In Months
67	48	227	218.5	8.5	3.74%	Aug-02	May-03	9
68	66	196	183.5	12.5	6.38%	Jul-02	Apr-03	9
69	70	228	221	7	3.07%	Jun-02	Apr-03	10
70	70	212	205	7	3.30%	Aug-02	Jun-03	10
71	42	205	185	20	9.76%	Sep-02	Feb-03	5
72	56	177	154	23	12.99%	Apr-02	Jan-03	9
73	55	165	156	9	5.45%	Oct-02	Apr-03	6
74	43	226.5	205	21.5	9.49%	Sep-02	May-03	8
75	46	250	244	6	2.40%	Mar-02	Aug-02	5
76	50	252	231	21	8.33%	Dec-02	May-03	6
77	50	217	191	26	11.98%	Jul-01	Jul-02	12
78	75	153	145	8	5.23%	Jul-02	Oct-02	3
79	72	207	201.5	5.5	2.66%	Mar-03	Jun-03	3
80	62	206	200	6	2.91%	Oct-02	Mar-03	5
81	73	181	173.5	7.5	4.14%	Nov-02	May-03	6
82	69	224.5	221	3.5	1.56%	Feb-03	Jun-03	4
83	70	142.5	140	2.5	1.75%	Aug-02	Oct-02	2
84	71	184	180	4	2.17%	Apr-02	May-03	13
85	56	173	165	8	4.62%	Feb-02	Dec-02	10
86	73	243	231	12	4.94%	Jan-02	Feb-03	13
87	78	233	223	10	4.29%	Oct-02	Jun-03	8
88	44	277	262	15	5.42%	Aug-02	Sep-02	1
89	44	142	135	7	4.93%	Apr-02	Oct-02	6
90	57	171	135	36	21.05%	Dec-01	Nov-02	11
91	72	229	224	5	2.18%	Aug-02	Oct-02	2
92	55	311.5	305	6.5	2.09%	Apr-02	Oct-02	6
93	48	171	152.5	18.5	10.82%	Jul-02	May-03	10
94	67	232	213	19	8.19%	Mar-03	Apr-03	1
95	56	216	204.5	11.5	5.32%	Sep-02	Apr-03	7
96	62	252.5	250.5	2	0.79%	May-02	Jun-02	1
97	86	214.5	198	16.5	7.69%	Aug-01	Jan-03	17
98	48	271	267.5	3.5	1.29%	May-02	Jan-03	8
99	72	219	202	17	7.76%	Feb-02	Aug-02	6

Table 1 – Positive Patient Results Using the Chang Method (continued)

	Age	Start Weight	End Weight	Change in Lbs.	Percent Change	Start Date	End Date	Time In Months

Table 1 – Positive Patient Results Using the Chang Method (continued)

	Age	Start Weight	End Weight	Change in Lbs.	Percent Change	Start Date	End Date	Time In Months
100	49	236	208	28	11.86%	Jul-02	Jan-03	6
101	49	230	223	7	3.04%	Feb-02	Sep-02	7
102	69	161	157	4	2.48%	Feb-02	Dec-02	10
103	72	156	152	4	2.56%	Oct-02	Jun-03	8
104	45	282	240	42	14.89%	Apr-02	Jul-02	3
105	74	170	156	14	8.24%	Feb-03	Apr-03	2
106	51	178	174	4	2.25%	Jun-02	Jan-03	7
107	45	230	228	2	0.87%	Jul-02	Sep-02	2
108	56	270	265	5	1.85%	Oct-02	Jun-03	8
109	44	194.5	190	4.5	2.31%	Jul-02	Jan-03	6
110	60	249	242	7	2.81%	Apr-03	Jun-03	2
111	57	230	229	1	0.43%	Feb-03	Jun-03	4
112	74	195	186	9	4.62%	Apr-02	Apr-03	12
113	44	221	200	21	9.50%	May-02	Mar-03	10
114	74	238	235	3	1.26%	Jun-02	Jul-02	1
115	74	147	143	4	2.72%	Aug-02	Jan-03	5
116	45	361	350	11	3.05%	Jul-02	Aug-02	1
117	68	209	195	14	6.70%	Nov-02	May-03	6
118	59	271	265	6	2.21%	May-02	Jun-03	13
119	73	233	228	5	2.15%	Sep-02	Nov-02	2
120	68	181	169	12	6.63%	Sep-02	Mar-03	6
121	51	257	251	6	2.33%	Aug-02	Nov-02	3
122	65	208	205	3	1.44%	Dec-02	Jun-03	6
123	62	227	223	4	1.76%	Jun-02	Apr-03	10
124	56	215	209	6	2.79%	Apr-02	Nov-02	7
125	81	203	198	5	2.46%	Feb-03	Apr-03	2
126	74	225.5	223	2.5	1.11%	Sep-02	Mar-03	6
127	72	266	254	12	4.51%	Sep-02	May-03	8
128	63	234	224	10	4.27%	Mar-03	Jul-03	4
129	61	186	171	15	8.06%	Jul-02	Jul-03	12
130	74	189	184	5	2.65%	Mar-03	Jul-03	4
Averages:								
	59.11	214.26	203.94	10.32	4.87%			5.94

Larry was very pleased with my program and wrote: "I am pleased with your recommendation to check my weight daily. It does work, and in two months I have lost about 17 pounds. On any day in which I notice that I have gained a pound or two I immediately work on it so that it will not make a home with me. This has also brought my blood pressure back to normal. Before this, it was beginning on an upward trend. I have now gained confidence that I will attain my desired weight and the important thing is that I know now how to maintain it satisfactorily."

Husbands and wives can follow my program in a joint effort, as illustrated by Judy: "Last year Dr. Chang told my husband and me that we needed to lose weight to improve our health problems. My husband was on the verge of being a diabetic. I started reading labels on everything I bought and we went on a low-sugar and low-fat diet. I started to gradually lose a few pounds. I also weighed myself every morning before I showered and recorded it on the calendar...when my clothes started to feel loose that made me feel very good...I have lost at least 14 pounds and am almost ready to buy a size smaller. I feel great. Thank you, Dr. Chang."

I was stunned by the successful results of this study. During my medical practice in the past twenty-seven years, I have always emphasized the importance of diet, exercise and weight control. In fact, I would ask each of my patients about their diet and exercise regimen

Table 2 – Negative or Neutral Patient Results Using the Chang Method

	Age	Start Weight	End Weight	Change in Lbs.	Percent Change	Start Date	End Date	Time In Months
1	57	233	239	-6	-2.58%	Sep-02	Nov-02	2
2	76	226	226	0	0.00%	Apr-02	Aug-02	4
3	69	222	226	-4	-1.80%	May-02	Jul-02	2
4	76	207	208	-1	-0.48%	Oct-02	Feb-03	4
5	55	218	223	-5	-2.29%	Jan-03	Apr-03	3
6	57	152	153	-1	-0.66%	Aug-02	Oct-02	2
7	57	184	184	0	0.00%	Jul-02	Apr-03	9
8	40	185	185	0	0.00%	Oct-02	Mar-03	5
9	62	166	172	-6	-3.61%	Apr-02	May-03	11
10	58	180	184	-4	-2.22%	Dec-02	Jun-03	6
Averages:								
	60.7	197.3	200.0	-2.70	-1.36%			4.8

almost every time they came to see me. This approach resulted in no more than a 5% success rate. For the past year, I've been using the daily weight monitoring method on my patients. As you can see from above, it's been tremendously successful. You may wonder whether there is something magical or special about me that makes this method work. I want to dispel that notion.

I instructed a patient of mine in the daily weight monitoring method in September 2002. He returned two months later with a successful weight loss of 5 pounds. A few days later his wife (also my patient) told me she, too, lost 5 pounds in two months. I asked her how she did it. It turned out that her husband told her about my program. She weighed herself every day when her husband did. This illustrates that secondhand instruction also works.

Another example where the spouse lost weight following the directions I gave to my patient was in this account by Jonathan: "I followed Dr. Chang's directions for weight loss for four months and I lost 6 pounds. Previously I had been gradually gaining weight. I believe the main key to success (besides reduced fat intake) is weighing daily. This causes you to react immediately to any gain before it gets out of hand. By the way, my wife lost 8 pounds during the same period by following these directions."

To support my findings, let me introduce the National Weight Control Registry study. Researchers Drs. Rena Wing and James Hill wondered if anyone succeeded in long-term weight loss. If so, how did they do it? Drs. Wing and Hill founded the National Weight Control Registry in 1994 to study weight loss and weight loss maintenance strategies of people who succeeded in losing weight and keeping it off. To be eligible for the study, individuals had to have maintained a weight loss of at least 30 pounds or more for at least one year.

The researchers recruited over 3,500 subjects from all over the nation. They follow these people yearly with questionnaires regarding weight loss and weight maintenance behaviors. This study has been ongoing for over six years. At the time the study was published the average weight loss reported was 60 pounds!

Drs. Wing and Hill found three behaviors in a vast majority of the National Weight Control Registry subjects which, they concluded, accounted for the success of the group. First, these subjects engaged in high amounts and a wide variety of exercise, averaging sixty to ninety minutes per day. The most common exercise was brisk walking. Second, they were on low-fat, low-calorie diets. And third, these subjects reported regular self-monitoring of weight, many of them on a daily basis.

This study and my study are convincing proof that daily weight monitoring is not only effective, but is essential for successful long-term weight loss. From a risk-benefit analysis, there is absolutely no risk involved and the benefits are great. It is also inexpensive both in terms of time and money. It only requires a few seconds a day to weigh yourself, and the only cost is a reliable scale for those who do not have one.

The reason that daily weight monitoring works is that it empowers you to stay in charge of your own destiny. It puts the responsibility of your weight and your health in your hands. You do not need to rely on anyone else to tell you what to do. This is probably what accounts for the tremendous enthusiasm and success my patients experienced following this program.

Helene, who welcomes the responsibility of taking care of her own health, wrote: "The bottom line is that I cannot lie to myself about what I'm eating. The afternoon visits to the snack machine do count. The run to McDonald's because 'I'm too busy' does matter. I matter. With my daily appointment with the scale, I take care of me daily."

Frankly, it is mind boggling that almost all of the weight reduction programs discourage people from weighing themselves daily. For those of you who are still not convinced that such a simple approach will work, I challenge you to give it a try. That is the best way to find out. If it works for you, you will become a member of the elite club of less than 5% of the population who succeed in long-term weight reduction.

Remember, you have nothing to lose except weight!

Patient Testimonials

These are additional comments from Dr Chang's patients who have benefitted from the Chang Method of daily weight monitoring and weight loss.

BL: Retired Air Force *(lost 14 pounds in five months)*

"I weigh myself every day. If I put on a few pounds, I know I have to exercise more that day. I try to walk on my treadmill twenty minutes every day and watch what I eat. I am feeling much better about myself."

WE: Adult Education Teacher *(lost 4 pounds in ten months)*

"I have diabetes and high blood pressure, but have been able to avoid medication for the diabetes through exercise and weight control. The weight control is accomplished by weighing myself about five times a week on the average. Daily weighing lets me know if I ate too much in one day. If I have put on weight, then I have to watch what I eat closely for a few days until the weight goes down. This works well for maintaining my blood sugar readings and I am able to understand why my blood pressure readings are what they are. I believe the daily weighing helps me maintain a healthier lifestyle and makes me feel better."

HD: Higher Education Administrator *(lost 10 pounds in ten months)*

"After consulting with Dr. Chang, I implemented his advice to weigh daily, at the same time each day. This method inspires a daily awareness of my weight fluctuations and helps me to adopt a daily discipline, when necessary, to lose the extra few pounds that creep up over time.

"The method makes us aware that 'diet' is one of the

multiple factors that keeps us in a healthy state as we age. Over a period of ten months, I lost 10 pounds—the 10 pounds gained over time since my 40s. I am now 53. I appreciate his method and find it effective. This keeps the weight loss (2 to 3 pounds) manageable rather than requiring some complicated diet for another 10 pound loss."

JJ: Retired *(lost 6 pounds in four months)*

"I followed Dr. Chang's directions for weight loss for four months and I lost 6 pounds. Previously I had been gradually gaining weight. I believe the main key to success (besides reduced fat intake) is weighing daily. This causes you to react immediately to any gain before it gets out of hand. By the way, my wife lost 8 pounds during the same period by following these directions."

WT: Assistant General Manager *(lost 9 pounds in two months)*

"I am a single mother with three teenage children. I have always preached the importance of weight control to my children but recently found myself gaining weight. With my 40th birthday nearing and not feeling well either emotionally or physically, I turned to Dr. Chang at the suggestion of my fiancé. Since my visit to Dr. Chang in October, I bought a scale and religiously weigh myself daily. I don't allow the scale to govern my life but use it as a source to keep myself in check. There are days with great gains (2 to 4 pounds) and there are the days of small losses (1 pound) but I know with the knowledge I have now, I will be successful in my venture towards weight loss and a healthier lifestyle."

MM: Homemaker *(lost 8 pounds in ten months)*

"I have been experiencing weight gain due to depression

from outside influences and a lack of exercise. After talking to Dr. Chang, I began walking five days a week on average for thirty minutes. I watch my fat and salt intake more now than before. I weigh myself once a day in the morning only. It helps keep me from overeating when an extra pound shows up."

SC: Registered Nurse *(lost 14 pounds in eight months)*

"I was skeptical when Dr. Chang introduced the daily weighing program. I felt it was not necessary especially since all of the diet programs I had been to in the past said weigh once a week. But I found that weighing myself daily gives me much more motivation to stick to my diabetic weight loss regimen. If I gain 1 pound I encourage myself to lose it by the next day. If I am the same weight or have gone down, I give myself a big pat on the back and encourage myself to continue. This plan has really worked for me."

SY: Occupation Not Given *(lost 5 pounds in six months)*

"I have always had a weight problem. I tried different kinds of diets and always got discouraged right away. Dr. Chang recommended that I try weighing myself every day. I bought a scale the next day and started weighing every morning. This has made a big difference. I'm very conscious about what I eat now. If I gain a pound, I watch what I eat to bring my weight down. If I lose a pound, I'm excited and try to keep it off. This has helped me to lose weight easily."

MB: Retired Registered Nurse *(lost 15 pounds in six months)*

"I think of myself as an intelligent person. But I was unable to lose weight successfully until Dr. Chang explained the importance of weighing every day! Along with this, I increased the amount of exercise I was doing, which allowed me to keep a close check on any weight fluctuation. These two things plus modifying my dietary habits assisted me in losing 15 pounds in just a few months."

EJ: Occupation Not Given *(lost 3 pounds in two months)*

"Daily weighing has helped keep my weight in check, especially during the holidays. I now feel in control of my weight and am confident that I can meet my weight loss goals."

JM: Housewife *(lost 3 pounds in three months)*

"I told Dr. Chang I thought I was gaining weight. He told me to find my comfort weight and write it down. I have lost weight because I weigh myself every day and I know how to gauge myself with my eating. It works!!"

MD: Caregiver *(lost 19 pounds in nine months)*

"I've been going to Dr. Chang since 1979. I went on his weight maintenance program in April 2002. At the time I weighed 177 pounds on the scale. Yesterday when I weighed it was 158. Physically I feel good losing that extra baggage. Here is my regimen: weigh yourself daily to make sure that you haven't put on extra pounds, cut back on your sugars and eat at least three meals a day."

LJ: Retired *(lost 7 pounds in eight months)*

"Dr. Chang's advice on how to lose weight really worked for me. He said to weigh myself every day, cut back on my portions of food daily and then maintain the weight loss even if it was only a few pounds. The important thing was to maintain the loss."

XJ: Occupation Not Given *(lost 5 pounds in six months)*

"The regimen of stepping on the scale every day has

been helpful. If the scale shows a gain you can be extra careful with what you eat that day, maybe also adding more exercise, such as a second walk or a bike ride. These actions will probably ensure stabilization or a slight loss to show the next day. I find that very encouraging. If you think you are eating carefully for a week, then get on the scale to see a gain, it is discouraging. A week's effort down the drain is a lot worse psychologically than one bad day.

"It is important to weigh at the same time every day, either in your birthday suit or in the same clothing. This routine eliminates potentially misleading results; for example, weighing yourself before breakfast one day and after breakfast the next is an inaccurate comparison of weight, as is weighing nude versus weighing dressed.

"When I injured my leg and couldn't do my usual exercise for several weeks, I got discouraged about my weight and stopped weighing daily. Bad idea. Now that I'm back out hiking and biking, I'm on the scale every morning, hoping that vigilance will help me drop a few (or a lot!) of pounds."

KM: Acupuncturist *(lost 6 pounds in six months)*
"I find Dr. Chang's program very effective and easy to follow. It does not require taking medication or any special regimen. I take daily weight readings before going to bed and another reading as soon as I get up. I walk about half an hour daily in the evening in the mall, where it is a safe and warm, pleasant environment.

"Of course I eat a lot of vegetables, fruits, fish and take vitamins daily. Try to cut down on sweets, bread and too much rice. Thank you for your excellent program."

LW: Real Estate Broker *(lost 6 pounds in three months)*
"Knowing that I would weigh myself every day with

the goal of maintaining my weight challenged me and made me aware of what I was eating and the exercise I needed. I am now sure that I can lose the weight that I want and keep it off as long as I make it a personal daily goal."

IK: Office Manager *(lost 6 pounds in six months)*

"Through the guidance from Dr. Chang, I have embarked on a program to lose weight and improve my health. I have followed his instructions on weighing myself daily. This has been a tremendous help. Those extra pounds can add up very quickly when you are not keeping track. I can make little daily adjustments in my food intake to make sure I stay on track. Thanks to Dr. Chang's advice and encouragement I am losing weight and keeping it off."

GD: Administrative Assistant *(lost 50 pounds in ten months)*

"I lost 50 pounds on Weight Watchers. I've been at my goal weight for four months and feel that by weighing myself daily I am in control. If I weighed myself once a week, I could easily gain 5 pounds. If my weight is more than 2 pounds above my goal, I immediately decrease my points the next day."

HM: Housewife *(lost 20 pounds in eight months)*

"In the past, weighing only occasionally, I seemed to gain/lose continually. Since weighing myself daily, I find if I gain even half a pound, I am aware immediately and can take steps to keep my weight in check. Thank you, Dr. Chang, for your advice and care."

EJ: Retired Teacher *(lost 10 pounds in four months)*

"I have been practicing your suggestion of keeping my fat grams under 40 per day. Also I have weighed myself each morning—a necessary incentive for being ever watchful about foods consumed during the day. I feel one of the major ways to track a person's weight loss is to weigh each day at about the same time—without exception. Exercise is always a contributing factor to weight loss but because of my current back condition I am able to exercise very little, but still find myself losing weight—thanks to the daily weigh-ins and being careful with fat grams. Thank you, Dr. Chang."

HC: Priest *(lost 26 pounds in twelve months)*
"For many years I have weighed myself daily. I believe that it helps me keep my weight in check. Without daily monitoring I feel the pounds will start mounting up and I will stop being careful of what and how much I eat. While this is not the only thing I do for weight control, it's certainly a helpful tool."

MJ: Electrical Engineer *(lost 6 pounds in seven months)*
"Weighing myself each morning serves as both a reminder and a challenge to my goal of losing weight. When the reading on the scale is lower than yesterday, I feel satisfied and driven to lose more. When the daily reading is more than yesterday; I am challenged to make it up."

UB: Retired *(lost 14 pounds in six months)*
"I have been on this program for six months through Thanksgiving, Christmas and New Years. The first thing I do when I get up in the morning is to weigh myself with no clothes on. I have cut out most of breads, candy, cookies and ice cream. I really believe in this program."

HS: Claims Adjustor *(lost 4 pounds in seven months)*
"The bottom line is that I cannot lie to myself about

what I'm eating. The afternoon visits to the snack machine do count. The run to McDonald's because 'I'm too busy' does matter. I matter. With my daily appointment with the scale, I take care of me daily."

HH: Physician *(lost 11 pounds in five months)*

"Following your suggestion I am now weighing myself daily. This has been helpful to me for the following reasons: I know from day to day what my progress is. If my weight goes up the slightest bit, I can adjust my caloric intake right away. Monitoring my progress closely gives me confidence that I'm doing the right thing. I can keep close tabs on my progress and not wonder how I'm doing. There is a daily reinforcement that I'm being successful."

LD: Sales and Service Representative *(lost 17 pounds in two months)*

"I am very pleased with your recommendation to check my weight daily. It does work, and in two months I have lost about 17 pounds. On any day in which I notice that I have gained a pound or two I immediately work on it so that it will not make a home with me. This has also brought my blood pressure back to normal. Before this, it was beginning on an upward trend.

"I have now gained confidence that I will attain my desired weight and the important thing is that I know now how to maintain it satisfactorily."

NE: Executive Assistant/VP *(lost 12 pounds in five months)*

"I have tried many forms of weight reduction over the years but have never felt as 'in control' and inspired as I do following Dr. Chang's plan. Knowing that I will be stepping on that scale in the morning makes me very aware of exactly what I am eating.

"Although you asked me to try this regimen in October, I started and stopped several times and by January my weight once again soared out of control. On January 15, I finally began following your suggestions and lost 7 pounds in the first four weeks. I have now lost a total of 12 pounds.

"I am not (for a change) trying to lose all of my excess weight at once. My only goal is to weigh less on the last day than I did on the first day of each month. I feel better about myself than I have in years and if I only lose 1 pound each month, that's ok. At least it won't be a gain!"

TM: Homemaker *(lost 4 pounds in five months)*

"Having a program you can live with and follow is of utmost importance. The first thing each morning I weigh myself and set my goals for the day."

TA: Retired *(lost 14 pounds in two months)*

"I have lost 14 pounds in two months just by keeping my total fat grams under 40. I do not exercise but do stretching exercise for my arthritis. This has been the easiest weight loss program I ever had. I plan to use it the rest of my life. Weighing every day is very important because you can see the results and the progress you make."

JD: Housewife *(lost 14 pounds in six months)*

"In September of 2002, Dr. Henry Chang told my husband and me that we needed to lose weight to improve our health problems. My husband was on the verge of being a diabetic. I started reading labels on everything I bought and we went on a low-sugar and low-fat diet.

"I started to gradually lose a few pounds. I also weighed myself every morning before I showered and recorded it on the calendar. It gives you an incentive to watch what and how much you eat. I cut back on servings and made nice progress. It was slow but the results showed. When my clothes started to feel loose that made me feel very good. Even when we go out to eat I still watch what I eat. I also choose from the basic food groups and stop eating when I feel full. No snacking in between meals. I have lost at least 14 pounds and am almost ready to buy a size smaller. I feel great. Thank you, Dr. Chang."

FJ: Builder *(lost 13 pounds in eleven months)*

"I get out of bed each morning and the first thing I do is step on the scale. Day by day I know what my weight is and if it goes up a pound I am aware that I should maintain my intake to avoid any more weight gain and adjust to lose the pound. For the last six months my weight has maintained itself within a 4 or 5 pound range."

EM: Retired *(lost 3 pounds in four months)*

"I have been dieting for fifty years, sometimes very successfully, but I always gained the weight back. I am a good example of a yo-yo dieter. Dr. Chang's daily weighing has been a success for me because it puts me in control. It is a lot easier to lose 1 pound than 5. I have learned which foods make me gain and also make me retain water. It seems to make me more conscious of every thing I put in my mouth. Here's to more weight loss."

GR: Retired *(lost 10 pounds in six months)*

"Since October 2002, I have weighed myself every morning. This has proved to be an excellent incentive for me in my attempts to lose weight. Since February 2003, I have lost 10 pounds. I find if I weigh every day I get an early warning of the slightest weight gain. I can then make an immediate adjustment in my food intake. Weighing every day also provides me with a personal challenge to maintain any loss."

JP: Registered Nurse *(lost 12 pounds in seven months)*

"Weighing myself every day has made me more aware of my body and how it can change quickly. It has helped to keep me on track and reach each goal I set for myself."

MO: Retired *(lost 13 pounds in nine months)*

"My husband and I weigh ourselves every day. We find it rewarding as a way to maintain our weight loss. We also find that if we weigh more frequently we watch ourselves closely and end up losing more weight. This program really helps."

Index

A

abdominal obesity 1-3
adrenaline 39-40
aerobic exercise 33, 36, 41
aerobic riders 34
Antihypertensive and Lipid Lowering
     Treatment to Prevent Heart
     Attack Trial (ALLHAT) 55
Amarillo, Texas 80
amputation 3, 50
angiotensin-converting enzyme (ACE)
     inhibitors 54-55
angiotensin-receptor blockers 54
arthritis 26, 62
Atkins Diet 25

B

basal metabolic rate (BMR) 9
base line weight 13
beta-blockers 54
blindness 5
blood glucose 3
blood pressure 31-32, 37, 40, 47,
     52-55, 118
blood sugar 6, 19, 43, 45, 47
body mass index (BMI) 2-3
bread 25, 28

C

calcium channel blockers 54
Calorie Control Counsel 2
cancer 1, 39, 48
carbohydrates 25, 27-29
cardiovascular disease 1, 39
carotid artery 49

central obesity 2
cholesterol 26-32, 37, 39
chronic low back pain 59

D

daily weighing 11, 17-20, 32, 46, 53,
     55, 111, 113
degenerative joint disease 57
diabetes 1, 3, 6, 17, 38, 42-46
diet 8, 10, 19-20, 23-25, 27-31, 40,
     44, 46, 53, 56, 108, 112, 118
dieting 9, 11, 18, 21, 78
diet products 24
disabled 77, 105
diuretics 54-55
Doc Rock 96-98

E

elliptical trainers 34
Elvis Presley 96
energy expenditure 8-9
energy intake 8
every day weight monitoring 11
exercise-induced thermo genesis 9

F

"Fight or Flight" hormone 39
fat 3, 9, 13, 18, 20, 25-31, 40, 44, 58,
     112, 118, 120-121
fluid retention 11, 13
free fatty acids 3
fruit 10, 25, 28-29

G

gallbladder disease 1
gangrene 3, 50
glipizide 45
glucose 3, 42
glyburide 45

glycerin 3
goal 15-16, 20, 22, 27-28, 94, 96, 107, 110
Graves Disease 82

H

happiness 102-104, 106
HDL (good cholesterol) 39
heart disease 1, 3, 27, 31, 39, 42, 55
heredity 6
high-carbohydrate 25, 28
high-fat 25-26
high-protein diet 25
high blood pressure 1, 39, 46, 52, 55
hypertension 52-56

I

insomnia 40, 69-70, 72
insulin 3-4, 38, 42, 45
internship 86-89

K

karaoke 99
ketosis 26
kidney dialysis 5
kidney failure 4, 52
kidney stones 26

L

LDL cholesterol 26, 28, 31-32
low-carbohydrate 25
low-fat 25-27, 40, 44, 121
low-fat diet 27

M

martial arts 101
Mercy San Juan Hospital 64, 74, 96
metabolic syndrome 1

metformin 43-46
moderate-fat 25, 28-29
moderate-fat, high-carbohydrate diet 28
moderate-protein diet 25
monitoring your weight every day 11
monounsaturated fats 29
mountain oysters 83
Mr. Choi 79, 82-84

N

National Cholesterol Education Program 29
National Institutes of Health 29, 54
National Weight Control Registry 40, 111, 120
nerve endings 5
New England Journal of Medicine 43, 45
nonsteroidal anti-inflammatory medication 57
Nordic ski machines 36

O

obesity 1, 3, 6, 8, 24, 33
omega-3 fatty acids 29
Ornish Program 27
oral hypoglycemic agent 45
osteoarthritis 1, 57
overweight 1, 2-3, 10, 27, 43, 53, 110

P

pasta 25, 28
pelvic tilt 59
Pima Indians 6
Polyunsaturated fats 29
Pritikin Program 10, 27
protein 25, 27-28

R

respiratory problems 1
retinal disease 4
rowing machine 34

S

saturated fats 29-30
scale 12, 18, 20-22, 109, 121
Sha Na Na 97-98
sleep apnea 1
smoking 48-50, 90-91
StairMaster 36-37
stair steppers 34
stationary bicycle 33
straight-leg-raising exercises 58
stress 27, 36, 39, 57-58, 60-61, 64,
       67, 69, 72, 74, 76, 88
stroke 1, 3, 39, 42, 48-49, 51-52, 55
sugar 6, 19-20, 25, 42-43, 45, 47, 118
sulfonylureas 45
surgery 9, 50, 57, 60, 62, 75

T

Tai Kwon Do 100
thermic response to food 9
thermostat 8, 16, 109
tolbutamide 45
Transient Ischemic Attacks (TIA's) 49
transverse abdominis muscles 61-62
treadmill 33-36
triglycerides 1, 3

U

uric acid 26
USDA Food Guide Pyramid 28

V

very-low-fat diet 25, 27
vitamin E 27

W

water pills 54
Weight Maintenance Mode 12, 14-
       15, 21-23, 26, 107, 109
Weight Reduction Mode 15, 17, 21-
       22, 26, 85, 88-89, 107, 110
Weight Watchers 16, 28

Y

yo-yo diet 11

Z

zinc 27
Zyban 51

About the Author

Henry K. Chang, M.D. is an internist who has practiced medicine in Carmichael, California since 1976. He has treated tens of thousands of patients over this period of time. As a passionate proponent of exercise, good nutrition and prevention of disease, Dr. Chang has created a revolutionary weight loss method incorporating—yes, a simple five-second daily routine. After developing and applying his innovative method, Dr. Chang has had unparalleled success: a whopping 93% of his patients have lost weight—and are keeping it off!

This book is based upon Dr. Chang's original study of 140 patients who followed his new, simple weight loss plan and achieved dramatic results. Thrilled with his patients' success, he couldn't wait any longer. He knew his break-through method must be shared with others who are struggling with excessive weight. So he wrote this book.